Jenni~

Keep living.

Sharing it!

Yo~ Kate Woening

Praise For Kate Horning

"Kate has a refreshing enthusiasm for healthy living and innovatively balances nourishing foods with life's pleasures."

Rachel C. Miller, MS, RD, LD

"Kate is a beautiful person inside and out. Her knowledge, enthusiasm and passion to inspire others to live a healthy and active life is contagious. I admire her as a professional and as a friend. I wish we lived closer, so she could cook for me and then we could train together!"

Katie Uhran is the owner of
She Rocks Fitness in Houston, TX

Live It. Share It.

Healthy Living Redefined

Live It. Share It.

KATE HORNING

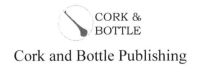

Cork and Bottle Publishing

Healthy Living Redefined: Live It. Share It. Copyright © 2014 by Kate Horning. All rights reserved. Printed in the United States of America. No part of this book may be used or reproduced in any manner whatsoever without written permission except in the case of brief quotations embodied in critical articles and reviews. For information address Cork and Bottle Publishing, PO Box 910616, Lexington, KY 40591.

Cork and Bottle books may be purchased for educational, business or sales promotional use. For information please write: Special Sales Department, Cork and Bottle Publishing, PO Box 910616, Lexington, KY 40591.

Book website: http://healthylivingredefined.com
Publisher website: http://corkandbottlepub.com
Author website: http://katehorning.com
Facebook: http://facebook.com/SimplyNutritiousbyKate
Twitter: http://twitter.com/nutritiouskate

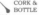
CORK &
BOTTLE

Cork and Bottle Publishing
Lexington, KY

FIRST EDITION
Published 2014

Library of Congress Cataloging-in-Publication Data is available upon request.

ISBN 978-0-615-96652-6

10 9 8 7 6 5 4 3 2 1

For my incredible parents who have been there supporting me every step of the way throughout this journey. I am so grateful for every bit of love, encouragement and guidance you have given me.

And for the chef who inspired me to look at food a little differently – thank you.

For Those Fighting Childhood Obesity – $1 of every book sold will be contributed from the author's royalties to help fight childhood obesity through health and nutrition education.

"Insanity: doing the same thing over and over again and expecting different results." – Albert Einstein

aka dieting.

Contents

II
PRACTICE

Book Progression

This is a non-technical manual on how to create a healthy lifestyle. It is comprised of six sections, each representing a step in the process of building a practical, sustainable lifestyle. I use my own lifestyle as a guide. The first five sections are method. The final section is practice and brings it all together into a simple 28-day guide you can use to create your own healthy lifestyle.

Step 1

Review Where You Came From

Step 2

Use Experience To Process What You Learn

Step 3

Mindset Is A Critical Skill For Maintaining A Lifestyle

Step 4

Reflect Often

Step 5

Convert The Most Effective Lessons Learned Into Habits

Road Map

An Example Of What A Healthy Lifestyle Looks Like

A Quick Note

1. This not a diet book. This is a better-than-a-diet book. If you're searching for a "lose-weight-fast" plan, I can't help you.

2. You already know what you should do. I may introduce you to a few new things, but the fundamentals are the fundamentals.

3. I will introduce you to a new way of looking at things and give you some framework to build your own healthy lifestyle.

4. The only person you can change is yourself. You have to be willing to try.

5. Remember, health is about the journey so don't forget to enjoy the ride.

How To Get The Most Out Of This Book

Draw all over it! Take notes, cover it with stickies, and highlight the hell out of it! Treat this book like a workbook or better yet, an idea book. I've left big margins so that you have plenty of room to make it your own. I want you to use this book as a resource and regularly come back to the material again to see how it relates to your own experiences.

The goal is to get you to think differently and to look at the world in a new way. I'm sure you've read tons of books on health and dieting with each one telling you that they have the solution to your weight loss or health issues. I'm not going to do that.

I want to open your eyes and make you think in a way that helps you create your own healthy lifestyle – one that fits your needs. One tailored to your own hectic, crazy, wonderful life. For that, I'm going to practice what I preach and share my story, ideas, and thoughts to inspire you to think more about your own.

At the end of each section, you will find a summary of the important points made in that section entitled "Create Your Own Healthy Lifestyle". If you wish to review what you have learned, these serve as quick references or reminders you can reflect on.

One valuable tool that I share in this book is the 28-Day Road Map. This is intended to help you reflect on your own health each day. It is not a set of instructions. It does not tell you what to do. It's simply a type of journal for where I am in my healthy lifestyle, the thoughts I reflect on, and the way I approach food daily. It is what it says it is – a simple road map you can use to create your own.

Remember that this is not a destination but a journey for you to continue travelling over the course of your life, changing and shaping your healthy lifestyle along the way. Read each section completely and then stop to think about it for a while. You'll be tempted to rush ahead to the next section, but try to resist.

Make some notes for yourself. Mark places you want to revisit or sections that may become clearer with further reading. After you've had a chance to digest what you've learned, you should then continue to read.

Some Thoughts On Why I Wrote The Book

There is so much information on health and nutrition out there that most of us can feel overwhelmed. It's too complicated. We all know what to do; we just don't know how to process the information. It's both the blessing and the curse of the technology-driven world we live in. We have all the information in the world at our fingertips and no guide on how to process it. If you want to know the latest on health, nutrition, dieting, fitness, or anything else, just Google it.

What I have written is a guide on how to process this information, focusing on the positives like food and life while getting away from the negative mindset of dieting and deprivation. I wanted to share the sort of ideas and thoughts my friends and I discuss over dinner and a nice glass of wine. I've always found that sharing our insights on what works for us—and equally on what doesn't—is how we learn and inspire each other best and with that in mind, I've laid down the framework I use to approach my own healthy lifestyle.

The goal of this book is simple – to serve as inspiration for you to shape your own path. By its very nature, it's a work in progress. If I've learned anything, it's that life is learned best by living.

Epiphany Moment And The Absence Of Common Sense

When did I decide this book should be written? It was the senior year of my dietetics program in college. I'd spent the previous four years studying to become a dietitian and was looking forward to getting out there and helping people.

In addition to what I was learning at school, I had been getting more involved with the "locavore" scene by working at the local co-op and getting to know the farmers who provided the fresh produce. I was also trying to expand my knowledge by reading books like Kris Carr's recently-released "*Crazy, Sexy Diet*," and became very conscious of using whole, natural foods.

The assignment was pretty straightforward: design a three-day meal plan for a diabetic patient.

No worries. I've got this. I spend time making sure the patient gets a variety of whole, natural foods and vegetables, with a strong focus on fiber and healthy fats to balance the patient's blood sugar. I'm proud of my work.

When I got the paper back, the green smoothie I recommended for breakfast on day one was circled in red with the following handwritten note in the margin:

"This is too complicated. Too difficult to measure and count. I suggest using foods that are already in the system. I recommend fiber cereal and skim milk for a healthy breakfast."

"WTF?!" Are you serious?

Healthy Living; *noun*

Healthy Living is the act of enjoying a holistic lifestyle that acknowledges the importance of taking small steps to develop habits that form the foundation for personal happiness, well-being and success.

Aside from the prevention of disease, we recognize that mental clarity, energy and a state of feeling good are important in increasing our productivity and value in both our professional and personal lives.

In short, healthy living makes us the better at the one thing we have to do every single day – LIVE.

A Path Of Obsession Some Call Passion

Step 1 – Review Where You Came From

Rebellion At Thirteen

At the age of thirteen, I was starting to think about my health for the first time as well as how food was actually affecting my body. After doing some reading and researching, I was reconsidering the idea of eating meat. I had never really enjoyed it and thought that by removing it from my diet, I could focus on eating more vegetables and plant-based foods that I knew made me feel good.

I was sitting at dinner one night, staring at the piece of meat on my plate and trying to figure out how the heck I could get out of eating it. Then it occurred to me that I would just tell my parents I wanted to be a vegetarian! After all, vegetarians don't eat meat!

After thinking about it for a few days, I finally plucked up the courage to bring it up. My mom, being the supportive (if slightly controlling!) mother that she was, surprisingly agreed but told me that I had to do more research and really understand my choice. She made me write a book report on why I thought becoming a vegetarian was the right decision and how I would go about replacing the protein and other nutrients that I needed to be a healthy, active, growing girl.

So off we went to the local book store, leaving with a stack of books that I just couldn't wait to get home to read. For the first time in my life, I found myself passionate about something and couldn't wait to embrace it. I may not have realized it at the time, but I had just taken the first step in my journey towards creating my own healthy lifestyle.

Lesson Learned: Your health is a journey not a destination. Start today!

High School Activist

My passion for learning about health and nutrition continued into high school. I started to get involved in as much as I could to learn about how health and nutrition really impacted our bodies. I enrolled in every nutrition-focused elective I could and got my first job at a health club to be around like-minded people.

Nutrition class became my obsession and as time wore on, I developed a super-close relationship with my teacher, who encouraged me to spend as much time as I could helping the other nutrition classes. I also shared my passion for healthy cooking by helping to teach other students how to cook a little better during the hands-on kitchen segments of class.

My ignited passion led me to get involved with the school lunch program and I began working to get healthier options in the school lunches. I talked about the effect of what we were putting on kids' trays and encouraged the school to put healthier options in the soda and vending machines.

Lesson Learned: Sharing your passion makes you want to learn more.

Starting To Think I Can Make A Difference

By my senior year of high school, I had become quite involved with the PTA school lunch program. Much to my surprise, I was asked by the Ohio State School Board to represent students across Ohio about the school lunch program and how it was affecting childhood obesity.

I don't remember much from that day. I was just so nervous and excited and couldn't believe that anyone wanted to hear what I had to say. It was kind of a whirlwind. I got up in front of a huge group and after some early jitters, I do recall realizing how passionate I was to share what I was learning with others. I genuinely felt that what I had to say could make a difference in people's lives but at the time, I wasn't able to fully express my passion as I would have liked. I remember the food they provided at the event was a little less healthy than I expected. I questioned some of the packaged granola bars and low-fat snack options and knew that this was really not the healthiest way to eat. There had to be a better way.

Sitting on the panel, I was surrounded by a table full of adults. I listened to a lot of educated people talk about what they discovered through research and case studies. While slightly intimidated at first, I knew that I needed to share my experiences from school. Listening to the other panelists, it struck me that it was no good to just have nutritional education in the board room – we needed it in the schools. Students were choosing pizza, pasta, and hamburgers over salad. They were throwing away the fruit and vegetables on their plate. And it was all because they simply didn't know any better.

I talked a lot about milk consumption and how students were drinking low fat or chocolate milk over water with lunch. I explained how they chugged sodas that they had purchased from the hallway vending machines during class. I shared how I noticed many of the high school girls thinking that chemical-loaded diet soda was a better option than water. I focused on how making small changes to lunch menus while increasing education on how to choose healthier options at school could really impact students' health both in and out of school.

Lesson Learned: Don't let your fear control you. Share your passion, it might inspire someone.

Getting Dumped Messes Up The Relationships That Matter

Up until the last few months in high school, I was on the path to eating more healthily while changing my perspectives on food. I had been a vegetarian for a few years and was eating a plant-based diet, but I placed no limits on how much I ate. I was an athlete and a teenager, so I was pretty much hungry all of the freaking time.

I also had the privilege of growing up in a family that had a very healthy relationship with food. We sat at the dinner table to eat every single night and from what I can remember, I never heard my mom say the word "diet" in front of me. I believed that as long as I ate "healthy," I could eat whatever I wanted. I had a great relationship with food and embraced eating without thinking twice.

Towards the end of my senior year of high school, that all changed. I had a boyfriend who dumped me completely out of the blue for a girl that—in my crazy mind—seemed to be skinnier, prettier and cooler than I was. This was the first time in my life that I began to doubt my lifestyle and how I was eating. I felt the need to control things in my youthful desire for boys to like me.

I swapped out some of my large portions of veggies and pasta for salad with low-fat dressing or dry packs of tuna. My go-to "diet" lunch at school was often an English muffin with a tablespoon of peanut butter. I would skip breakfast for the first time in my life and started eating breakfast cereal bars, thinking that they were a better option than my favorite homemade oatmeal with brown sugar and berries.

I started watching how much I ate and controlling my portions so much during the day that I would end up ravenous by my evening babysitting job. Being away from home, I would eat whatever they had in the house, which was often not healthy at all. It was my first experience with any yo-yo dieting and although I didn't experience anything too dramatic, my relationship with food became very restrictive and—more worryingly—exceptionally unhealthy.

I was struggling with what I put into my body and with how it was making me feel. I began counting calories and incorporating more packaged foods due to the convenience. I was taking all of my intuitive knowledge about how best to treat my amazing body and throwing it out the window because of what I was going through.

It was a stressful time.

Lesson Learned: Food is meant to be embraced not restricted. Trust yourself!

Calorie Counting, College And Soda. What Else Could Go Wrong?

I went off to college and decided to pursue my passion in nutrition by enrolling in dietetics at the University of Kentucky. I was really excited because we started our nutrition classes in the first semester and the desire to expand my knowledge had me almost skipping to class every day.

At this point, I was still struggling with my relationship with food and I was trying to find the "perfect diet." Almost immediately, we began to learn about counting calories, carbs, fat and protein. I was also learning about the latest food trends of the time which were very focused on low-carb, low-fat, and fat-free foods.

At school, we had to purchase software to calculate calories and learned about how they impacted our health and weight loss. I thought I could start counting calories myself as a way to more effectively control things in my life. At first, I would add my spinach salad with low-fat ranch dressing into the calorie counter software. It took quite a bit of time, but I thought that I was finally starting to get it right. I mean, this is what I was going to school for.

However, I discovered that it was easier to start incorporating packages into my diet because the calories were already calculated for you on the label. As an example, the back of the frozen dinner box had a controlled portion with the calories clearly defined for you. I would still be hungry and would grab pizza with my friends when we would go out at night. I would also eat in the cafeteria at school, but when I could control what I ate, I did it with packaged foods.

Of course, being away from home for the first time (coupled with being at college) led to a lot more partying. I joined a sorority and found that my exposure to large quantities of alcohol, late-night pizza, and endless junk food buffets increased dramatically. I started drinking soda for the first time in my life, and even though I knew that I wasn't treating my body well, I thought of myself as healthy.

This period was definitely the low point in the journey to creating my healthy lifestyle.

Lesson Learned: Sometimes you have to just learn it the hard way.

Healthy Made Me Feel Like Crap

By the end of my junior year of college, I was beginning to believe that I was finally figuring it all out. I wasn't partying as much. I was controlling my food intake. I was really watching my calories. I was going to the gym five, six, and sometimes even seven days a week. I was participating in high-intensity workout classes and eating "clean". I really thought I had it under control.

However, I was feeling worse than ever before. I started to get sinus infections and other random afflictions on occasion. I know this sounds lame but up to that point in my life, I very rarely got sick. My energy was low and I felt tired all the time. I blamed it on my schedule as a student or the occasional night out.

I tried to fix it with energy drinks, even though I knew they weren't good for me. It was what everyone else was doing so I figured, "what the heck." I felt the pressure to perform. I needed to get through studying, work, going out with friends, and still set a good example by looking the part of a dietetics student.

I was at the point where I was trying to figure out why I was feeling like crap. I believed I was doing everything exactly the way I was learning it in school. I was eating healthy, portion-controlled foods like egg white and spinach omelettes (with egg whites from a carton), spinach salads with fat-free ranch dressing, low-fat yogurt and fat-free cottage cheese with sugar-free granola, and frozen diet meals.

I thought I was following the rules and eating "clean" yet something wasn't quite working.

Lesson Learned: Diets don't work!

The Stress Of Perfection

As my journey continued, I began to realize that I was looking for perfection. I believed that everything would fall into place if I could just keep it together. I would feel confident in my body, have huge supplies of energy and feel amazing. If I just kept my portions in check, got at least one intense workout in daily, and stayed away from bread, wine, cheese, and sweets, I would be OK.

However, I never got to that point where I was OK. If I had a day where I didn't go to the gym, or where I went out for pizza and a beer with friends, I felt guilty and obsessed over it. The problem, however, wasn't the pizza and beer – it was the guilt. This regular guilty feeling would lead me time and time again into a cycle of self-destruction. If I would have pizza, I would have a cupcake, and then I would have ice cream and it would become a downward spiral from there.

The problem with this extremist mindset was that everything had to be "just so" or it would throw off my entire plan. All I had to do was get everything perfect and everything would work out from there. And if it wasn't for one seemingly trivial experience, I may have never transformed my mindset and found the path to creating my healthy lifestyle once and for all.

The gym that I went to while in college had a section available for student parking that was not owned by the campus. I would often take classes at the gym or get a work out in between my college classes and would always push it right down to the wire.

I had it down to a science. I would rush straight over to the gym, park in the student area where I was sure to find a spot and bust out my workout. Then I would move on with my day. That was until the student parking area changed its policies. It was no longer reserved just for students, and all of a sudden I couldn't find a place to park.

The first time, this meant I missed a workout session. I spent the rest of the day stressed and felt guilty for not doing what I was supposed to for my health. The next day, I was determined to fix the problem and find a spot. I cut class and rushed over to the gym.

There wasn't parking anywhere! I was a college student with limited funds so I avoided metered spots as often as possible. However, the only spot I could find was a ten minute walk from the gym and it was metered. I sucked it up and parked. When I got done with my workout, I ran over to my car and, sure enough, I found a ticket waiting for me. I was pissed!

This process was repeated over several days. I would try and find the right time to get a parking space, park in front of a meter five-to-ten minutes away and get a ticket. My workout classes were an hour long but the meters would only allow an hour of time.

I know what you're thinking. Why didn't you just find another gym? Don't you realize skipping college classes was a bigger deal than skipping a workout class? But in my mind at the time, I felt this need to be perfect, in shape, and healthy. I had blinders on to anything else. My stress was so high over this feeling of having to be perfect that I was in another downward spiral and not even aware of it.

The meltdown came when I ran out of the gym to find a boot on my car. The tickets had added up and I had almost gotten towed. I cried. I felt guilty, stressed and stupid all at the same time. Ultimately, I quit going to the gym and it would be months before I was able to regroup as the guilt and stress kept building up.

Although I went on with my life and eventually got back to my regular workout routine, it took me years of reflection to finally discover that I hadn't created a lifestyle but a forced routine. I always tell people that if you can't do it every day for the rest of your life, then don't waste your time.

And that is exactly the problem I created for myself. At the time, I knew what I was doing couldn't be sustained in the long term. I was forcing things into my schedule and striving for perfection instead of building a strong foundation to create a healthy lifestyle that worked for me. I saw health as an all-or-nothing approach and when something got in the way of that, I crumbled. What I know now is that moving my body every single day is so much more important than cramming in that forced, stress-inducing workout.

Lesson Learned: There is no such thing as perfection.

The Healing Power Of Whole Foods

As time went by, I began to develop headaches from stress. I never really got back into any sort of consistent exercise routine and I was still eating my calorie-counting diet. However, while complaining to a friend about my headaches, she recommended that I visit a chiropractor as this had brought her relief from similar issues.

I met a great chiropractor in town and really listened to what he had to say about getting to the root cause of health and nutrition.

This taught me to look at things a little differently. I shifted my perspective to a real-food diet and became passionate about looking for ways to incorporate more whole, plant-based foods into my lifestyle. Without even realizing it, I started to let go of packages and calorie-counting and began to embrace food again.

This first shift lead me to join one of their "sugar-free cleanses," which focused predominately on cutting out all grains and most forms of sugar (excluding berries and Granny Smith apples). Once the cleanse was finished, I was shocked by how much better I started to feel. I had more energy and felt so amazing that I wanted to learn more. I re-discovered my love of eating veggies but found that veggies alone were not enough. Since I was so hungry all the time, I started adding in rice and quinoa and began to experiment with a variety of other diets to see how tweaking certain things would affect my body.

Eventually, my experimentation brought me to a high-raw food diet. I stuck to this for a while but the lack of variety in my lifestyle meant that I got bored after a month. This resulted in a transition back to my vegetarian diet before I found my way onto a gluten-free vegan diet. This approach made me feel so amazing that I stuck to it (aside from the odd piece of good bread) for well over a year, which in turn forced me to recognize what an impact what I ate had on my health and quality of life.

Lesson Learned: Discover what works for you.

The Feeling That Something Is Missing

I spent the remainder of my college days tweaking, adjusting and expanding my new whole-foods, plant-based diet. I continued my vegan lifestyle but I was starting to experience a whole new stress – a stress to be perfect and to hold it all together once again.

I am a tad OCD by nature, but I know that I'm not the only one who feels this way at one point or another. I was so thrilled that I had finally discovered a lifestyle that I was thoroughly enjoying and embracing. I was learning all about organics and super-foods such as spirulina, chia, maca and chlorella. I started juicing and fell in love with green smoothies, buckwheat, and bee pollen.

However, I started to experience stress around this all-or-nothing approach. I preached the whole-foods, plant-based diet to my friends and family but I also emphasized that the most important part was finding a lifestyle that works for you. I did that for everybody else but crucially, I wasn't doing it for myself.

I still remember going to dinner at a friend's house and reminding them of my dietary choices ahead of time. The host made asparagus and mashed potatoes just for me to enjoy and when she brought out the plate, I noticed she had drizzled hollandaise all over the asparagus. She was so excited to see what I thought of it but I had to wait until she walked away to wipe the hollandaise off of the asparagus so I could eat it.

This is where everything finally clicked for me – I wasn't treating food as something pleasurable anymore. Instead, I had fallen into an extremist health-food mentality and struggled once again to hold together this "perfection" I had created for myself.

I found that what I was doing wasn't a sustainable lifestyle for me and it certainly wasn't a sustainable approach to healthy living. I had given up foods that I truly enjoyed and started to make food more of a fuel source that fit onto a cookie-cutter label.

I had been avoiding going out with friends just so I wouldn't have to eat non-organic food and if I did go out, I would try to find a slice of gluten-free vegan pizza while they all ate what they wanted. I would stress out if I ate something unhealthy or if I missed a day at the gym and I would constantly put myself down if I didn't drink my daily green smoothie or get enough sleep.

Even though I truly believed I was onto something good, I felt that there was still a piece missing in my own life as well as the lifestyle I was sharing with others. I kept thinking that if I could only discover how to sustain a stress-free healthy lifestyle in the long term that things would all fall into place.

Lesson Learned: You don't have to give up everything you love to be healthy. In fact, it's important to find pleasure.

Rediscovering Food And Seeking Holistic Healing

As ever, I wanted to learn more about health and nutrition so I took a job at the local co-op as a way to continue my healthy evolution. On my first day, the manager was making fresh mozzarella cheese from curd. Of course, I was an obsessive vegan at the time and I watched intently as he went through the whole process, explaining it to me as he went. Then, out of nowhere, he handed me a piece to try!

I was terrified. I didn't know what to do. One part of me felt that if I tried it, I would expose myself as a fraud but at the same time, I had just watched him make it from scratch. So, I went for it. I decided I couldn't pass up the chance and, much to my surprise, it was the most amazing mozzarella cheese I had ever tasted in my life. It was warm, and it was gooey, and it had this amazing salty flavor. It was like nothing I had ever experienced before.

That experience and others like it continued to shape the way I thought about food as an experience and a source of pleasure. I began to think more about what it meant to really embrace food. I would chat with the local farmers as they came into the co-op. They would invite me down to the local markets where I came to understand more about what it meant to eat seasonally. I discovered for the first time how mouth-watering a tomato tasted right off the vine on a summer day, as opposed to something lying on the shelf at the average grocery store in December. I began to see how high quality, fresh food could really impact flavor and how highlighting seasonal ingredients was essential to pleasure and enjoyment of food.

Naturally, this led me to try incorporating these discoveries into what I was already doing. With the experiences I was gathering from playing with whole-foods and seasonal ingredients, I decided to continue my education in nutrition from a holistic point of view. I wanted to keep expanding my knowledge and learn from other experts in different areas of thought so I enrolled at IIN (Institute for Integrative Nutrition) to get a broader perspective.

I wanted a "big picture" view and sought out conflicting

opinions to define and color my own thoughts. I learned even more about raw food and how it affects our well-being. I discovered how stress levels and sleep impacted upon my health and food choices, which I never thought about before. I studied a variety of dietary theories so I could further shape what I knew to be essential in creating a healthy lifestyle. I took it all in as I continued on my journey to look at health a little differently.

Lesson Learned: Food is best enjoyed when creating an experience around it.

Finding Pleasure In Food

With my new-found perspective on the impact of external forces on our health, my passion for food and cooking was revitalized. I was using amazing local ingredients from the local farmers' market and preparing them in a way that was all about pleasure and simplicity. Creating habits I could follow every single day became my new mantra.

I knew that improving my skills in the kitchen would make this quest more realistic so I started interning and teaching at a local health-focused culinary school where I could share what I was learning with others.

The owner of the school had attended the Natural Gourmet Institute in New York City, an establishment known for focusing on training chefs to view foods as health-supportive. Eventually, this led me to become a private chef and cook for larger groups of people. I was able to focus my efforts on changing their view of healthy food by making it about flavor, texture and experiences, making it all about how delicious simply prepared vegetables could taste.

Getting the opportunity to work with other talented chefs totally transformed my thoughts on food as an experience, both in terms of getting more pleasure out of food as well as the social aspect. I also began drawing inspiration from other cultures' approaches to food in relation to how they created experiences around food. My mindset was shifted to seeing food as something that you should find pleasure in, instead of something that should be controlled or viewed negatively. I became intrigued in the process of how food really affected our health, both nutritionally and from a holistic view.

Lesson Learned: Food should taste amazing. If it's not enjoyable, then don't waste your time!

A Healthy Lifestyle And Having Something To Say

Once I began teaching and sharing what I was learning with others, it didn't take long to discover that it was my true calling. I loved seeing people implement what I was teaching into their own lives so I started a business as a health coach and private chef.

I knew that no matter what I did, the focus of my new business had to be on teaching people how to live a little healthier. My own busy life had taught me that creating your own healthy lifestyle meant that it had to both fit in everything you needed while being sustainable over time. I had been shaping and fine-tuning my own healthy lifestyle for over a decade which gave me a great foundation but I was also aware that every individual person has different needs.

Since I often work 12-14 hour days, I realized that having a healthy lifestyle, eating right and taking time to move my body made me more productive and successful. I started sharing my insights and connecting with like-minded women who were very success-focused but struggling with sticking to their health choices as soon as life got in the way.

What follows is my approach to creating a practical and healthy lifestyle that will fit around your life rather than standing in its way. It's simple and straightforward and intended to be reflected upon. While my views are grounded in years of study, science and personal experimentation, I choose to share my thoughts in a more common sense approach. I believe that the role of books is to make us re-evaluate things we already know while making us look again at things we have forgotten on the surface but remember deep inside. If we don't occasionally take the time to reflect on these intangible truths, we run the risk of deceiving ourselves.

Companies invest millions in "top of mind" marketing. This is the idea that by keeping something in front of you often enough, you'll have their business or product on the top of your mind when you choose to purchase. It's a way to block out the competition by remaining connected. Take a page from their playbook. Invest in yourself! Take the time to reflect on your health. Keep it simple and make yourself "top of mind"!

Lesson Learned: Don't give up! You can live the life you desire!

Create Your Own Healthy Lifestyle

Review Your Life. What Works For You?

Some lessons from my own life:

- Your life is a journey not a destination. Start today!

- Sharing your passion makes you want to learn more.

- Don't let your fear control you. Share your passion, it might inspire someone.

- Food is meant to be embraced not restricted. Trust yourself!

- Sometimes you just have to learn it the hard way.

- Diets don't work!

- There is no such thing as perfection.

- Discover what works for you.

- You don't have to give up everything you love to be healthy. In fact, it's important to find pleasure.

- Food is best enjoyed when creating an experience around it.

- Food should taste amazing. If it's not enjoyable, then don't waste your time!

- Don't give up! You can live the life you desire!

Make It Your Own

Live It. Share It.

Step 2 – Use Experience To Process What You Learn

A 17th Century Samurai Changes My Life

A chef friend of mine had amazing knife skills that I really wanted to learn. I just loved watching him cook. He made it look so easy and peaceful. Relaxing.

When the opportunity to work with him came up, I took it. The job seemed simple: cook in front of twenty dinner guests and entertain them. Think Cooking Channel meets the Travel Channel with a healthy twist at a live dinner party.

All I had to do was cook, smile, and talk about food and health. My favorite things! How hard could this be? Little did I know what was in store for me.

We had a few weeks to prepare, so we hacked out a menu, talked about healthy cooking and did the typical things one does to get ready for a dinner party. Then he asks me the strangest question, "Have you ever cooked in high heels in front of people?"

"Ummm, no."

We were supposed to dress up as part of the dinner party. This meant no comfortable shoes, no chef jackets, no throwing my hair up. No hiding in the back kitchen. No making a mess. I was on a whole different playing field and hadn't thought about what that meant. I'm a messy cook on a good day. What was I going to do in a cocktail dress and heels in front of chatty dinner guests?

And so began my education. I'm impatient. Everyone knows that about me. I want to know it all and do it all instantly. I work hard, learn quickly and expect great things out of myself. I asked my friend to teach me to cook like he does; clean, graceful and with awesome knife skills. He laughs, and says, "OK."

The next day, I'm dressed in sweats, a t-shirt, and high heels. Cutting board in front of me, knife in hand. Over the next eight hours, I'm taught how to properly hold a knife and use it skillfully. Like boot camp, I'm constantly being told, "Wipe your board! Clean as you go."

I have to learn not to rush. Clear my mind. Avoid my more obsessive tendencies. Cut, stir, cook and plate calmly to avoid making a mess. Be aware of time as each dish is prepared. And most importantly, wipe my knife and board constantly.

I learned two lessons that day. Firstly, I'm impatient, often biting off more than I can chew. Secondly, heels suck.

My friend is encouraging. He says I did really well and I just need to practice. I feel overwhelmed, stressed and frustrated. I'm pissed that I'm not as good as he is, worried that I'll make an idiot out of myself.

I asked how I could become better. This is when I was introduced to the wisdom of Miyamoto Musashi, a 17th century samurai warrior that has since changed my life:

"Today is victory over yourself of yesterday. Tomorrow, victory over lesser men."

This means to stop thinking in terms of trying to keep up with— or surpass—everyone else. All you have to do is do a little better than you did the day before. Challenge yourself. Don't worry about everyone else or where they are. By focusing on improving a little each day, you will exceed everyone around you. Whatever your challenge, LIVE it every day.

I spent the next couple of weeks practicing. Not with succeeding or being awesome in mind. Not with being as good or better than my partner. Instead, I focused on making small, daily improvements. Competing only with myself. And you know what? I got dressed up in a black cocktail dress and four inch heels and I rocked that party!

The Secret

This was the real turning point for me. I began to see my whole journey in a new light. I realized that life was an experience; one that was reborn every morning, but rested on what was discovered the day before.

Like most, I had made it way too complicated and placed too many unnecessary expectations on myself. It was less like running and more like perpetually falling, afraid for the day I didn't catch myself. I'm not even sure who or what was defining my successes and failures, much less shaping my views on them. There was only one thing I was clear about – it wasn't me.

There is a transcendent yet difficult-to-communicate feeling of calm that comes from the realization that the only thing you can control is yourself. Living is interesting in that it has no destination, there is no sense of completion, and no possibility of perfection. You must simply live.

You can however, control what you do with each beautiful day. You can't control what others think about your actions. You can't control what others say. That's why focusing on your own growth will allow you to reach your greatest potential. Simply do a little better than you did the day before. That's the secret.

A little demonstration I like to use to illustrate the potential of doing just a little better every day is this: take a single penny and place it in your hand. Pretend that the penny is you. Now double the amount in your hand each day for just thirty days. The first day is the first time you double the amount. Do you know the result?

On the first day you are only worth $0.02.

By day 10 you are worth a whopping $10.24.

By day 20 you are worth a respectable $5,242.

And if you keep making steps each day, by day 30 you are worth over $10 million.

Try it for yourself. Take a piece of paper and write 1-30 on it. Start with a penny and then double that amount each day. You'll see what the power of focusing on small, incremental growth is about. At first you won't see much change. You may even feel the need to rush it. Don't. As the days go by, the results will get bigger and bigger and others will take notice. They will recognize the change in you, not because you were doing anything to meet their expectations, but because the growth inside yourself was significant enough to take notice.

That's how we make real changes in our lives. Small steps.

The Power Of Experiential Learning

Often, the most difficult thing to accomplish is the one most simply stated. It's overwhelming, looms over your head and creates paralyzing fear. Where do I start? What do I do?

Remember to take a deep breath and a single small step. You don't have to solve everything at once. You just need to spend time reflecting on it. As you grow, so will your understanding and ability to implement what you have learned.

I believe that experience is the greatest teacher of all, but we need structure and guidance to keep from going insane. Aristotle said it best,

"For the things we have to learn before we can do them, we learn by doing them."

The best method that I've come across for getting the most out of our experiences and really making them part of our growth is the "See One, Do One, Show One" method. This is a method of learning used in the military and in the medical field to teach hands-on skills in real time. It's a method to rapidly learn and develop new skill sets. "See One, Do One, Show One" is at the heart of my "Live It. Share It." philosophy.

For this method to work, there are a few things we have to accept:

1. You must be willing to get actively involved in the experience. This means you have to get your feet wet and get your hands dirty. Nothing will come out of life if you do not experience it. There will be highs and lows. You can reduce the chances of having lows by reading, taking classes, and working with a coach or trainer, but real growth comes from the experience. Don't be afraid.

2. Growth will come with reflection. Taking the time to reflect on your experiences, the things that you have learned, and the things that you are just discovering will allow you to better grasp the insights that will come to you.

3. Use what works for you and discard the rest. This isn't about becoming a parrot or one-size-fits-all. This is about adapting what works best for you from your own experiences.

Put simply "See One, Do One, Show One" is:

See One: *This is where we intellectualize information.* Be introduced to new ideas. Read as much as possible and often. Learn from experts, but also from friends and family. Work with a coach or trainer.

Do One: *This is where it becomes practical information.* Try it. Try what you are learning. Eat more greens. If you discover that you may have a wheat intolerance, try going gluten-free and see if it improves how you feel.

Show One: *This is where we take ownership of the information.* Show others what you are learning, especially how what you have discovered works for you.

Time To Simplify Things. Live It. Share It.

There are two things you can do to make your healthy lifestyle a success. Live it. Share it. I've intentionally repeated this phrase throughout the book. I've even made sure those four words were all over the cover. At its simplest, this is how you create your own healthy lifestyle – by living it for yourself, and sharing what you learn with others.

Living it incorporates the "See One" and "Do One" steps we have learned. If I were to give you a step-by-step plan to live your healthy lifestyle, this would be it:

Step 1: Reflect on what you have learned and what you are learning for a few minutes every day. I recommend writing it down. Make your health top of mind.

Step 2: Read something new every day or watch a new video, listen to a new podcast, etc. There is amazing, inspirational content everywhere!

Step 3: Focus on improving one small thing from the day before.

Step 4: Forgive yourself if you screw it up. Remember that it's about consistency and change over time.

Step 5: Live life. Find small pleasures and take care of yourself each day.

Sharing it incorporates the "Show One" step we learned. This step is extremely important and one that I believe most people underestimate. This is where you really make what you have learned your own and begin to see it in new ways. This is where mastery happens.

To teach someone something—or to share with them—you have to look at it from their point of view. You have to be able to answer questions from your own experience and why it works for you. You have to be able to describe how it has affected your life.

This makes it real. It deepens your reflection on the subject and makes you understand it in new ways. It gives you greater insight and allows you to learn new and greater things.

Sharing is also a great way to provide accountability for yourself. By sharing, you are proactively living your healthy lifestyle and making it a part of who you are instead of something to check off a list.

Sharing what you have learned does not mean stubbornly defending an idea. That stunts growth. It means to create a conversation that further opens each other's minds.

Finally, and let's be honest, we need support. Sharing your journey with a friend or loved one will help both of you when we reach the inevitable stumbles that accompany growth. We're not meant to grow alone.

Create Your Own Healthy Lifestyle

Learn To Live It. Share It.

- The only thing you need to do is be better than yourself of yesterday. Take small steps.

- There are only two things you need to do in order to ensure success in creating a healthy lifestyle:

1. Live It.

Live your life, get involved, reflect often and use what works for you.

2. Share It.

We are not meant to grow alone.

- Practice experiential learning: See One, Do One, Show One.

Change Your Mindset

Step 3 – Mindset Is A Critical Skill For Maintaining A Lifestyle

Create A Growth Mindset
For Yourself

The importance of mindset in creating a healthy lifestyle for yourself cannot be understated. It is one of two skills (the other being reflection) that you must develop to maintain a sustainable lifestyle. One could easily argue that mindset is the most critical skill to possess.

But what is "mindset"? We hear the term bandied about a lot by motivational gurus and life coaches but a clear understanding remains elusive. By definition, mindset is the established attitude that we hold about something. Unfortunately, this leads you to believe that there are a different set of rules, guidelines or thought processes for everything you want to accomplish or change for yourself.

This doesn't seem right to me. If one looks closely, there are common traits shared among successful and inspiring people we admire. Typically, we distill these down to concepts of positive or negative. However, everyone—you and me included—possesses a bit of both. With this in mind, why do you think that intelligent, success-minded women struggle with how they see themselves, especially as it applies to health, beauty and their bodies? What mindset do we really need to achieve a successful healthy lifestyle for ourselves?

I began toying with the idea that if there were so many variations of "mindset" for each area we wanted to succeed in, what were the common themes or overlap? Looking at analysis of case studies for successful entrepreneurs, elite athletes and best-selling authors, I noticed the following:

Be positive.

Love to learn.

Be proactive.

Seek out challenges.

Find enjoyment in what you do.

Become self-motivated.

However, I couldn't escape the realization that if I already possess many of these traits—and have succeeded in other aspects of my life professionally—then why can't I do the same when it applies to my health? What am I missing?

These thoughts led me to the conclusion that there must be a core concept that I was overlooking. This is when I stumbled upon the work[1] of Dr. Carol Dweck, the Lewis and Virginia Eaton Professor of Psychology at Stanford University. Dr. Dweck has spent the past several decades conducting research on motivation and achievement, examining why so many highly intelligent students consistently fail to live up to their "potential", while others achieve in spite of the challenges presented to them.

Her work challenges widely held beliefs on intelligence, how we perceive ourselves and our ability to succeed. In her writings, she explains how students' theories on their intelligence or their mindset define what goals they choose to pursue and how these effect their adaptive or maladaptive achievement patterns. This creates the base for a complete "meaning system". In other words, how we perceive intelligence, and how we acquire it, will define how we see ourselves and our perception of what we can achieve.

She presents two competing views: a fixed mindset and a growth mindset. With a fixed mindset, intelligence is viewed as predetermined and unchanging – you're either smart or you're not. With a growth mindset, intelligence is associated with gaining knowledge and applying it. If you work hard, you can gain more for yourself.

If confronted with a difficult or challenging situation,

individuals with a fixed mindset will tend to avoid the situation and seek out opportunities that guarantee a higher rate of success. They have decided they don't have the necessary intelligence to succeed at that task.

Individuals with a growth mindset however, tend to view challenges as something they can overcome. They see intelligence as the result of hard work and are more likely to understand that "mastery is a process that takes place over time and with prolonged effort."

It's important to note that her research focuses on how the students saw themselves. She was intrigued by how many of the more accomplished students would shy away from challenges and fall apart in the face of adversity, while less skilled students would rise to the challenge and become motivated with setbacks. Many of the more skilled students expressed self-doubt in their abilities and questioned themselves. The students who saw challenges as something to overcome rarely showed such behavior. The good news is that when the fixed mindset students adjusted their perception, they learned that knowledge through incremental growth showed dramatic changes in their ability to overcome challenges.

Her work leads me to conclude that successes in other areas of our lives do not necessarily translate into success in our efforts to create a healthy lifestyle. We may have a fixed mindset. We're not dumb, hopeless or helpless; we just have to change our mindset.

The true effects of having a fixed mindset were very poorly understood until recently. Under a fixed mindset, we are predisposed to believe that we don't have what it takes, rendering conventional forms of encouragement completely pointless. Haven't we tried so many times before?

Unfortunately, many of us view our health as a pass or fail scenario. However, the truth is that successfully creating a healthy lifestyle is not found in the destination but in the journey, the looking, the learning and the growing. This can be achieved by shifting to a growth mindset. How is this accomplished? Live it. Share it.

As we learned previously, small daily steps are important for both creating and succeeding in your own healthy lifestyle. By simply improving and reflecting upon one thing from the day before, you encourage a series of small successes. Each subsequent success builds on the one before, helping you realize that challenges can be overcome through incremental growth. This will increase your self-confidence and self-reliance. As each new success brings you the benefits of living a healthy lifestyle, such as increasing energy, improved mood and motivation, new opportunities for growth will sprout in other areas of your life as well.

Having a bad day? Reflection and learning from your experiences, as well as daily self-improvement, create an inherent margin of safety. A better way to describe it:

Small steps keep you from big mistakes.

Your inevitable setbacks will be minimal, and you will be able to overcome them with continued daily effort.

If you are stuck in a fixed mindset, making the shift to a growth mindset may seem difficult. Sharing with a friend, loved one or even total stranger will help give you the "push" factor necessary to make lasting change. Sharing doesn't mean preaching or lecturing. It can be as simple as going for a walk with a workout buddy, sending a friend a new recipe you discovered or inviting a girlfriend at work to a new fitness class.

As I'm writing this, I've made plans to join a girlfriend this afternoon for a hot yoga session at a mutual acquaintance's studio. Who knows, maybe later this evening we'll grab a glass of wine and chat about what's going on in each other's lives. Remember that it's all about living – not diet and fitness obsession.

If you use social media, I encourage you to share via your

favorite platform. What are you doing to create your own healthy lifestyle? What works for you? What goals are you setting? Build some support and accountability for yourself!

Use the hashtag #liveitshareit on Twitter or Instagram and I'll make an effort to respond to as many posts as I can. Together, we can support each other.

Ask The Right Questions

In order to get what you desire, you have to ask yourself the right questions. It's important to take the time to do this properly. When you are taking time to reflect on yourself in the morning or evenings, focus on what you want to get out of life.

To get started, take out a sheet of paper and ask yourself some important questions. Take the time for personal reflection before you answer:

1. What do you really want? Do you want to feel good? Do you want to live longer? Do you want to look good naked? Be honest with yourself.

2. Describe what your ideal healthy lifestyle would look like. Keep it realistic. Save the eating chocolate cake every day fantasy and instead, focus on what works with your life. No one knows you better than you do.

3. If there was one thing you could do better today than you did yesterday, what would that be? Avoid dramatic statements like "eat healthier." Just choose a single, small, actionable item.

Now take the time to share your questions with someone else. Help them find their answers while sharing your own. Support each other.

The Philosophy Of Healthy Indulgence

There will be pleasurable experiences in your life that you do not want to give up for your lifestyle. Maybe you enjoy the delicious fat dripping off of a Carolina pulled-pork sandwich. Maybe you love the decadent silkiness of butter frosting on a chocolate cupcake. Maybe a food is culturally important to you and you don't want to trade fond memories of your childhood for restriction and deprivation. This is where the Philosophy of Healthy Indulgence comes in:

It's OK – in its proper place and proper context. The idea is to look at food differently. If you enjoy—and I mean truly enjoy—the experience of rum-raisin ice cream, then have a small scoop on occasion. However, make sure that you have a mindful experience while you eat it. Sit down and savor each bite. Make sure that it's the best tasting ice cream you've ever eaten and not some cheap thrill. Reflect on why you enjoy it so much and let it bring a smile to your lips.

Then move on. Don't over think it. Don't stress about it. Don't say to hell with it and have another bite, or grab a pizza or any other type of self-destructive behavior. Relish the experience and then get back to living your healthy lifestyle.

The Formula For Weight Loss

The formula for weight loss is simple. It is provided in this book for one simple reason. To make you stop thinking about it. Read it and move on.

$$Pr + E = WL$$

Where Pr = Portion reduction, E = Exercise and WL = Weight Loss

How much weight you lose with will be determined by what you eat and any mitigating illnesses you are currently experiencing. However!

WL ≠ H

Weight Loss does not equal Health

Does this mean that health is not about weight loss? Of course not. Our bodies are smart. They don't want to be fat. They don't want to be sick. Given the right circumstances, they will make every effort to correct themselves.

Diets don't work because diets don't give our bodies what they need. With diets, you can lose weight; in fact almost all of them are effective for weight loss for a short period of time. However, weight is a measurement and like all measurements, it is often misunderstood.

What we are really saying is that we want more energy. We want to look good. We want to live longer. Those things are not defined by weight. When our goals are what we genuinely desire, weight loss happens naturally. We've given our bodies what they need to take care of themselves.

Life Gets In The Way Of Health

Let it go. Living a healthy lifestyle is about living. That means living it every day. Don't stress when things get in the way or fall through. Just accept Robert Burns' wisdom,

"The best laid plans of mice and men often go awry."

Did you have going to the gym on your to-do list today only for a meeting to run long. Don't worry about it. Don't try to cram it in or reschedule it tomorrow. All you're going to accomplish is an increase in stress for the next day. Instead, go for a walk or take a few extra minutes when you're reflecting at the end of the day. Keep in mind, life is about living and a healthy lifestyle isn't about your to-do list. Just do the best you can and move on.

1. Dweck, Carol. *Self-theories: Their Role in Motivation, Personality, and Development (Essays in Social Psychology)* Psychology Press, 2000

Create Your Own Healthy Lifestyle

Create The Right Mindset For Yourself

- Create a Growth Mindset. Embrace incremental growth to overcome your challenges.

- Live It. Use small daily steps to build a series of successes that build upon the day before.

- Share your journey, successes, and challenges to give yourself the "push" to succeed.

- Share It. Give yourself a support network and create accountability for yourself.

- In order to get what you desire, ask yourself the right questions. What do you really want?

- You don't have to give up foods that you find pleasurable, but you do have to keep them in the right perspective.

- Weight loss does not equal health. If you create a

healthy lifestyle for yourself, weight loss will be a natural part of getting healthier.

- Don't forget that life is about living. If life gets in the way, don't let it stress you out. Simply move on.

- Daily reflection and self-improvement create a margin of safety so that you don't have to fear setbacks.

Learn To Think

For Yourself

Step 4 – Reflect Often

Through Reflection, We Grow

As I mentioned previously, there are two key skills that you must acquire to help you develop and sustain your healthy lifestyle. The first is the right mindset. The other is taking the time for reflection.

Reflection means to apply serious thought or consideration to a subject. It is the practice of thoroughly investigating and exploring what you are learning through your experiences.

Throughout this book, you will notice that I mention daily reflection quite a bit. Taking the time to think about things should be a consistent part of your healthy lifestyle and a habit in its own right. When you think about your health on a daily basis, it allows you to be more aware and have more mindfulness about the decisions you make in your day.

You do not have to spend hours of deep scholarly thought or put yourself into a meditative trance to accomplish this. Simply spending 10-20 minutes in the morning or winding down at the end of your day is sufficient. I typically spend a few minutes in the morning writing an inspirational quote or two in my gratitude journal or focus on my experiences while doing some yoga. In the evening, I may read a few chapters from a new book or visit some of my favorite cooking blogs.

During this time, I think about how I'm doing, how I feel or what I want to accomplish. Knowledge and understanding are built upon your previous experiences and new insights can be gained during moments like this. It's also a calm time for me as I shut out all external distractions and spend a little time in my own head.

If you spend as much time as I do reading books, you will discover that writings on subjects about philosophy, spiritual growth, and the arts (areas that typically take a life time to master) commonly have a recommendation for a period of reflection. Creating a healthy lifestyle is just one such art or skill. It's not mastery that we are seeking, but instead the ability to apply what we learn to our daily lives.

Notice that I am not recommending that you only practice self-reflection. While exploring your thoughts and emotions as you create your healthy lifestyle may be important, reflection on what you are learning about health, fitness and nutrition is vital too. This will allow you to simplify and wrap your head around any overly-technical or confusing aspects. Unfortunately, most of the material on health and wellness is unnecessarily complicated. Remember, the goal of your reflection is to simplify and enhance your own understanding of what you are trying to achieve.

Leonardo da Vinci himself said:

"Simplicity is the ultimate sophistication."

In a nutshell, this means that true understanding comes when you are able to clearly and simply state an idea. Now, that doesn't mean everyone else will understand. They need their own time to reflect. Learn to think for yourself.

To give you an idea about the sorts of things I spend my time reflecting on besides myself, here are some recent thoughts.

Body Weight Really Doesn't Change That Much

The human body is an amazing thing. It will do everything in its power to correct itself where possible. If it thinks you are starving, it will slow down its own metabolism. If it thinks it is in a time of plenty, it will create fat stores for another day. The problem comes in when the body doesn't know what is right and wrong. It doesn't have a healthy baseline to start with.

We are designed to survive and thrive. In truth, we can live on almost anything. While we may be designed for the natural world around us (and function optimally in that environment), we can also survive off of chemical-laden "food."

Over the centuries, this has allowed us to thrive as a species. We excelled at adapting to hunting, gathering, famines, droughts and anything else Mother Nature threw at us. But now, we're a victim of our own success as food is relatively plentiful. Distribution is such that we can pretty much get whatever we want.

This has caused us to become confused about our bodies. However, our bodies are a little more straightforward about the issue; if you eat fast food or other processed crap, your body accepts this as its normal diet. It doesn't know any better.

So, it fights to maintain the weight it associates with its primary food source. In other words, eat junk and your body will fight to stay fat. Diet or no diet, it just thinks in terms of feast or famine. And how do you break the cycle? You've got to give it a new base line.

Reset your body with new habits, starting with whole, natural foods and a predominantly plant-based diet. After it realizes it has a new primary fuel source, it will adapt. We're cool like that.

We Whip Our Own Asses

The guy sitting in a manufacturing kitchen reminiscent of a laboratory, adding a new chemical to increase the shelf-life of the latest GMO-based product isn't trying to kill you, at least not intentionally. He's just trying to solve a problem so that he can collect his paycheck – how do I keep this loaf of bread on the shelf for as long as possible?

Somewhere along the line, he stopped thinking in terms of flour, yeast and water and started thinking in terms of sales and distribution. It's not his fault though – we do it to ourselves. Money makes the world go round and there is something to that whole "supply and demand" thing. If we keep demanding convenience in a plastic bag, someone will provide it for us.

Surprised by the rise in gluten allergies? Up until a few years ago, most people had never heard of celiac disease and now it's widespread. Have you ever checked out the gluten-free options at your favorite restaurant? We did it to ourselves.

We wanted quick and easy bread – preferably white with none of that "whole-grain" stuff. Someone smelled a dollar and started changing the way we grew wheat. Then someone else changed the way we milled wheat. Then someone else changed the way we baked bread and so on.

At this point, it's debatable whether it's even accurate to refer to these products as bread. Wheat definitely isn't the same, and flour barely has anything resembling wheat in it anyway. I could talk about this issue for hours but the end result is this: our bodies don't like whatever this new wheat substitute is.

Eventually we have to learn our lesson.

We're Not All Doctors And They Don't Even Get It

I understand that this is complicated stuff. I also know that it's often difficult to translate complex problems in simplistic ways, but we have to try. No one wants to admit that we have no idea what we're talking about, but that really is the case.

The terminology we use for food, health and nutrition are better suited for clinical scientists than the rest of us. Even those trained in how to read and understand the studies being conducted aren't getting it. According to a 2012 Medline survey of 29,025 physicians across the country, 42% of male doctors and 32% of female doctors were overweight or obese.

We need to make every effort to explain health and nutrition in practical, common sense ways that we can apply in our lives every day.

When Did I Become A Lab Rat?

I often wonder if anyone finds it strange that we now seem to require a nutrition label before we decide to eat something. It seems that the same process scientists use when experimenting on rats has been applied to how many of us select our meals. At least the lab rat didn't pick it for himself.

How have we become experimental test subjects for food manufacturers? I've studied nutrition for most of my life and I couldn't tell you what half of those unpronounceable chemicals are. I'm not sure that many can. We pretend that we know what all of that stuff on the label means but truthfully, we have no clue.

Diet systems built on labels are even worse. They create number systems to rate how healthy a particular food is in order to make it easier for us to decide what we should be eating. However, if it needs a number for us to recognize that it's good for us, isn't that already saying something?

Today's Good For You Is Tomorrow's Bad

It never fails. Today's super-food is tomorrow's cancer-causing agent. Our knowledge about the world around us is always growing with the only consistent factor being change.

You must continue to develop and reflect on what you're learning. A lifestyle is meant to be practiced for your entire life. This means you have to keep evaluating and re-evaluating what you learn. Compare it to what you already know and see if you discover any new insights or changes in your perspective.

In short, a healthy lifestyle is less about what we are eating today and more about how we approach what we eat and what we do. Is there a good way to deal with the inevitable fact that today's healthy could be tomorrow's unwholesome? The answer is yes and you may have heard that it's "the spice of life."

Variety is vital to creating a healthy lifestyle. While eating whole, natural foods is essential to getting the most out of the human body, this does not mean that you should focus on super-foods only. Eating a variety of whole, natural foods creates a built-in flexibility that will give us the best defense against health trends or changes in what we know.

We Don't Eat Carbs, Proteins Or Fats

We eat rice, chicken and olive oil. Thinking in terms that don't really mean anything to us is not going to help build a healthy lifestyle. We often intellectualize these terms but don't really have a way of translating them into the real world. It's difficult to grasp through the lens of daily experience.

If I were to ask someone about protein for example, they will immediately reply "meat". It's how they translate the concept of protein into something they can touch and feel in their everyday lives. But what about the protein found in vegetables?

I believe that thinking about what you should eat in the way that you actually eat them makes it more real and practical. It makes more sense to say, "I'm going to have some rice with greens and a little chicken for dinner tonight." I can see it, touch it, smell it and taste it. This is why I focus on whole, natural foods.

There is no confusion about what a vegetable is except maybe a tomato!

Create Your Own Healthy Lifestyle

Reflect On What You Learn

- Reflection is the practice of thoroughly investigating and exploring what you are learning through your experiences.

- Reflect daily both in terms of self-reflection and with regard to your thoughts on what you are learning.

Things to think about:

- Body weight really doesn't change that much.

- We whip our own asses.

- We're not doctors and they don't even get it.

- When did I become a lab rat?

- Today's good for you is tomorrow's bad.

- We don't eat carbs, proteins or fats. We eat rice,

chicken and olive oil.

The Six Habits Of Healthy Living

Step 5 – Convert The Most Effective Lessons
Learned Into Habits

Habits Are The Rock A Lifestyle Is Built Upon

In order to create a long term, sustainable, healthy lifestyle, your efforts must be converted into habits. Habits are routine behavior that are repeated regularly and occur unconsciously. In other words, they're just something you do without thought. To decide what habits I should focus on, I turn to the 80/20 Principle.

If you are unfamiliar with the 80/20 Principle from the writings of Richard Koch or Tim Ferriss, it can be summed up as follows for our purposes:

20% of your effort will produce 80% of your desired results.

Conversely, the remaining 20% of your results often take 80% of your effort.

For example, eating well, regular exercise and reducing stress can get you to your ideal healthy body. You will look and feel good, and it requires consistent, yet minimal effort on your part. However, if you want to become an elite athlete, drop to nearly non-existent body fat, or run an ultra-marathon, you better be prepared for the blood, sweat and tears required.

Habits are what form the foundation of a healthy lifestyle. Consistent, repetitive, unconscious patterns of the fundamentals prepare you for success in your professional and personal life. As you get healthier and live better, your energy and motivation will grow. You will discover that you like the way you feel and may want to accomplish things in your life you never thought possible. That ultra-marathon is not out of your reach, it simply requires the first step. Develop habits.

Rome Wasn't Built In A Day; Neither Are Habits

It takes, on average, between one to two months to transform action or thought into habit, and there are a few things you can do to help ensure they develop.

1. Have a clear goal for your habit creation.

2. Like we have learned previously, small daily steps are key.

3. Live It. Build up to the habit you want to create. Don't feel you have to be perfect immediately. Start with where you are and remember that the only person you have to compete with is yourself. Focus on changing one thing about yourself at a time.

4. Share It. Tell someone about what you are doing. Create some accountability and support for yourself.

5. Look for a trigger. I recommend using your daily reflection as a way to trigger the development of a health-related habit.

6. Patterns are important. I have found the best way to accomplish this is to reflect daily on my health and consciously practice my target habits for three to five days straight. I will then take a break from thinking about them for a couple of days. This does not mean that I do not attempt the action; it just means that I don't make it a focus of my thoughts.

By following this method, you can let everything sink in and give your brain a chance to process your new habits on a subconscious level. I will then repeat this process and focus on the activity or thought for three to five days and then take a break for a couple of days before returning to it again over the full period of a 28-day cycle. If necessary, I'll repeat another 28-day cycle until it sticks.

For example, if I want to up my daily water intake (goal), I may draw eight circles on a sticky note in the morning as I'm reflecting on my health (trigger). Throughout the day, I'll then place a check mark inside one of the circles when I drink a glass of water (small steps). I'll use this method to ensure that I drink enough glasses of water for several days, and then I'll skip writing it down for two days (pattern).

I'm still attempting to drink plenty of water throughout the day, but I'm just not being as anal about counting them during those two days. I'll get back to writing it down again as I reflect on my health each morning and repeat the process. At first you'll be focused on making sure you're checking off each glass of water you drink, but after a while you will be like, "Yeah, yeah, I know."

That's when it will shift from conscious effort to unconscious habit. You probably won't drink exactly eight glasses of water each day after the habit is formed, but you will drink plenty of water throughout the day and that is what is important.

One thing I do want to mention is that developing habits is not the same as becoming obsessive. Leave some flexibility in your goals to take into account the randomness of life and don't chastise yourself if you miss a habit on any given day. Creating a lifestyle for yourself is about living, not developing self-destructive behavior. Remember, you can always revisit your habits and work on maintaining them if you ever feel that you're getting away from them. It's OK! It happens to me ALL the time.

Six Habits Of Healthy Living

After hundreds of hours of research and reflection, not to mention over a decade of personal experimentation, I have distilled the most effective 20 percent of effort down to six habits that produce over 80 percent of the desired results for healthy living. In other words, these are the core habits that need to be developed for a healthy lifestyle. These are the Six Habits of Healthy Living:

1. Dump Soda, Drink Water

2. Move Your Body

3. Eat More Greens

4. Track It

5. Lose Packages, Learn to Cook

6. Create Rituals

At first glance, you may be tempted to say, "Duh.", but don't fall into that trap. Like most things that are simply stated, they require consistent reflection to get the most out of them. As an example, Hippocrates' summary of the way we should eat is brilliant in its simplicity, but requires thought and reflection to make it your own:

"Let food be thy medicine and medicine be thy food."

For the following habits, I have intentionally chosen to explain them briefly. While they may be intellectualized, the true benefit of developing these habits can only be realized through reflection and by putting them into practice. What I can share with you is that making these changes and incorporating these habits will change the way you feel. Your palate will change and you will find more pleasure in food. Your energy will increase and you will have the stamina to achieve greater things for yourself. Your mood will change and you will find yourself happier and more engaged with the world around you.

This is something I can't teach you so much as guide you to experience for yourself. In the next section, namely the 28-Day Road Map to Create Your Healthy Lifestyle, I will go into more detail and show how I reflect daily on the habits below. I've listed them in the order in which I will focus on them.

Dump Soda, Drink Water

I've listed this habit first because it is the one that is going to have the greatest immediate impact on your body. We need to drink. We are hard wired to consume liquids in order to survive. However, what we drink is the single most effective way for us to abuse our bodies.

Liquids are the easiest way for us to introduce myriad chemicals, sugars and pollutants into our bodies. You would never eat a cup or two of sugar piled on your plate, but it's easy to consume that same volume in a matter of minutes if it's dissolved into a soda or sweet tea.

This applies to all forms of drinks. We were designed to drink water. Anything else can be considered a drug. Be aware of what you put into your body!

Make it a habit to drink plenty of water throughout the day and to be consciously aware of what the ingredients are of any other liquid you consume.

Move Your Body

We are not designed to be sedentary. Human beings were designed to move. This does not mean going to the gym for thirty minutes and spending the rest of the day sitting in front of a computer, TV or in the car. I mean MOVE!

Make it a habit to walk, stretch, do squats at your desk, whatever you can but move consistently throughout the day.

Eat More Greens

Dark leafy greens are some of the most nutrient-dense, natural foods on the planet. Incorporate more of these into your daily diet as you can. The boost in energy alone is phenomenal.

As a rule, eat more plants. Make it a habit to get at least 75% of what you eat from plant-based foods.

Track It

Tracking promotes reflection. It lets you see where you have been and where you are going. What you track is dependent on your goals. You may want to track your mindset in a gratitude journal or what you are eating in a food diary.

Regular reflection on what you're tracking allows you to better understand what you're learning while also acting as a motivational tool. Tracking also helps you meet your goals quicker as you increase your awareness of your efforts.

Make it a habit to create a journal or diary on the goal you are focused on and to reflect on it daily.

Lose Packages, Learn To Cook

Packages contain manufactured foods that mimic the whole, natural foods you should be eating. If it didn't grow in the ground, grow on a tree, swim, fly, or walk, then it's not food.

Cooking is a life skill we should try to develop. It doesn't require mastery. You don't have to be a chef, but you should be able to make as many of your meals as possible at home. This will allow you to get the most out of the whole, natural foods that are the foundation of a sustainable, healthy lifestyle.

Make it a habit to avoid packaged foods whenever possible. Learn to cook.

Create Rituals

Small daily rituals are the fabric that holds our lives together.

They are the experiences that make life worth living. Rituals also create patterns that improve the chances of developing habits for our healthy lifestyle.

Making a nice dinner and sitting down at the table with friends and family increases the chances of enjoying cooking. Taking a moment to appreciate the quiet of early morning (while enjoying a cup of tea) makes the experience desired and easily repeated.

Make it a habit to create small rituals in your day. You'll be amazed at how quickly you'll learn to love your healthy lifestyle when each new habit is as pleasurable as the last.

Create Your Own Healthy Lifestyle

Learn To Make Habits

- 20% of your efforts produce 80% of your desired results. Conversely, the remaining 20% of your results often require 80% of your effort.

To develop habits you need:

- A clear goal.

- Small steps daily are crucial.

- Focus on changing one thing about yourself at a time.

- Share what you are doing with someone.

- Look for a trigger.

- Patterns are important.

Reflect daily on the Six Habits of Healthy Living, the

core habits that need to be developed for a healthy lifestyle.

- Dump Soda, Drink water

- Move Your Body

- Eat More Greens

- Track It

- Lose Packages, Learn to Cook

- Create Rituals

28 Day Road Map

To

Create Your

Healthy Lifestyle

An Example Of What A Healthy Lifestyle Looks Like

Introduction

I've mentioned this in the beginning of the book, but it's important to repeat it here. The 28-Day Road Map is intended to help you reflect on your own health each day. It is not a set of instructions. It does not tell you what to do. It's simply a type of journal for where I am in my healthy lifestyle, the thoughts I reflect on, and the way I approach food daily. It is what it says it is – a simple road map you can use to create your own.

Follow these guidelines to get the most out of this section:

1. Use this section for daily reflection.

2. Read each day completely and then stop to think about it for a while. You'll be tempted to rush ahead to the next day, but try to resist.

3. Make some notes for yourself. Mark places you want to revisit or sections that may become clearer with further reading. After you've had a chance to digest what you've learned, you

should then continue to read.

4. You will probably find it difficult to apply everything you learn immediately. That's OK. Continue to revisit the 28-day Road Map every few months to get something new out of it.

5. Remember to share what you learn with friends, workout buddies, coworkers and family.

Below I have outlined what you will find in each day. Enjoy, and good luck with creating your own wonderful, amazing healthy lifestyle!

Breakfast

Upon rising, start your day with a big glass of room temperature water with the juice of half a lemon, followed by a cup of green or herbal tea and then breakfast.

This month, we're going to cut down the gluten (a commonly consumed ingredient in the morning) so it's time to hop outside the box and rethink breakfast. Some of my favorite options to start the day include a big green smoothie, sautéed greens with a fried egg, rice, oats, a frittata and even an avocado with scrambled eggs and hot sauce.

However, if you often find yourself running out the door in the morning (and eating on the run is not something I'd recommend) overnight oats, hardboiled eggs, and baked sweet potatoes are a busy person's breakfast BFF.

Lunch

Load up at least 50 percent of your plate with raw veggies (mixed greens, spinach, broccoli, carrots, tomatoes, cauliflower, cucumbers) and then top it off with steamed or sautéed veggies, quinoa, a homemade veggie burger, beans, legumes, tempeh, sauerkraut, baked sweet potatoes, and whatever else you like.

If you want to include a lean meat, limit it to just 25 percent of your plate and for dressing, dump the prepared crap and just finish your bowl off with a little olive oil, lemon juice or apple cider vinegar, and a pinch of Celtic salt. And if you'd like a little more flavor, add some hummus to give it a chickpea kick as well as a nice creamy texture!

Snack

For the next few weeks, I want to focus on nutrient-dense meals and limited snacking. Filling up your body with lots of fresh vegetables should help keep you full and happy in between meals, but if you find yourself hungry, reach for a few (10-12) raw almonds, some raw veggie sticks and hummus, Mary's crackers and guacamole, or a green smoothie.

And if you're craving a little pick-me-up by the time mid-afternoon hits, incorporate some tulsi tea for a little immune system and energy boost!

Dinner

Dinner should be similar to lunch. Start off with a base of raw or cooked greens (I love collards, kale, spinach, and arugula) and then top them off with whatever you like, the key being to keep your portions in check. You're more likely to metabolize food during the day when you're active than at night as our bodies need to focus on repair rather than digestion while we sleep. So slow down and savor your meal, eat until you're full and then relax!

Following dinner, it's time to unwind with a cup of herbal tea.

Dessert

Since this program is all about loading up on greens and nourishing our bodies, we shouldn't really be craving sweets and dessert. If, on occasion, you do have a craving that simply won't go away, I suggest a cup of herbal tea and a square of dark chocolate or one date or dried fig with a little raw almond butter to satisfy those urges.

Self Care

Self-care is essential throughout this program and in creating a long-term healthy lifestyle. Be kind to yourself, get plenty of sleep and start to take small steps each day towards better health.

Wake up and start your day off with a smile, gratitude, and some deep breathing. Savor your tea and then take a few minutes to move your body. On each day of the program, I will ask you to schedule one self-care activity. Whether it's getting a pedicure, a massage, taking a bath, curling up with a good book, or going for a long walk, you deserve to make yourself a priority!

Plus, if you're trying to lose weight, putting the focus on pampering yourself and living it each day will get you to your goals much faster than restriction and punishment, trust me!

Move Your Body

Movement is essential to both good health and weight loss. I want you to shift your mindset from going to the gym "X" number of minutes per week and instead, start simply moving your body daily. Need some inspiration? I have provided a daily tip to encourage you to move that little bit more.

Share It

At the end of each day I include a fun little reminder to share your lifestyle with others. Look for #liveitshareit

Day 1

Dump Soda, Drink Water

Welcome to day one of your transformation. For the next 28 days, we will be focusing on taking small daily steps to create a long-term, sustainably healthy lifestyle, while gently detoxifying your body.

Today's spotlight is on getting rid of soda (and all sweetened beverages for that matter) and bumping up your water intake.

If you're not already aware, soda is absolutely detrimental to your health in every way and yes, diet soda is just as bad. From the amount of sugar destroying your immune system (increasing your risk of diabetes and heart disease) to cancer-causing caramel coloring and artificial flavors to phosphoric acid (which contributes to osteoporosis, aging, and reproductive issues), soda is simply not worth the devastating effects it has on your health.

Soda also has a tremendously negative impact on the amount of glucose circulating in your bloodstream, otherwise known as blood sugar. A well-balanced blood sugar level is crucial to overall health and well-being as it regulates your hormones, triggers your body to burn stored fat, and increases your metabolism to help you lose weight.

When we drink soda, there's no fiber to slow down the absorption of all the sugar into our blood stream, leading to immense blood sugar spikes. This in turn causes an insulin burst followed quickly by a crash leaving you irritable, tired and craving more sugar.

Diet soda, on the other hand, is full of sweetening chemicals and it tricks your body into thinking that you have consumed sugar. However, diet soda lacks the calories that normally accompany sugar and it throws off your body's ability to know how many calories you actually need to be satisfied. This leads to over-eating and the resulting blood sugar spikes leave you worse off than if you had just had a regular soda.

Diet or regular, soda is not something we should be putting into our bodies if we're looking to create a healthy lifestyle. Instead fueling our cells with water is the key to long-term health.

When making the swap from sugar-laden beverages, hydration with plain H2O can get a tad boring. To combat this, try freshening things up by adding citrus fruits such as lemon, lime, and orange slices to your water. I also love adding herbs such as basil, mint, and even lavender to my water for a little extra flavor.

You can also use sparkling water as a nice fizzy option. The sweet and delicious taste of herbal teas are a great occasional addition as well. When choosing tea, however, it's very important to look for low-caffeine or caffeine-free choices like white or some varieties of green tea (save caffeine for the morning and stick to just one or two cups). Kombucha tea is also a fun alternative to water and makes for a great Healthy Indulgence.

To make sure I'm getting my eight daily glasses of water, I like to keep a tally. Pick up a journal or sticky note pad and make an effort all week long to track your water intake. I like to draw eight little circles and put a check mark in each circle as I down a glass of H2O to keep me aware of what I'm actually drinking every day. Once you get in the habit of drinking more water, it will come easily and you'll find yourself becoming more aware of when you're actually thirsty!

Here's Your Game Plan For Day 1!

Upon rising, start your day off with a mug of warm water with the juice of half a lemon and a small pinch of cayenne pepper. Sip that down followed by a cup of tea and then breakfast.

Wherever you go today, park a little further away and give your body a little extra movement!

Breakfast: Day 1

Keep breakfast simple this morning with a green smoothie.

Throw one small apple (cored), half a frozen banana, two handfuls of spinach, and half an avocado in the blender with water and ice to reach desired consistency!

Lunch: Day 1

For lunch, load up your plate with a big base of mixed greens and pile on raw veggies, a hardboiled egg, and a quarter cup of cooked quinoa, dressed with a drizzle of olive oil, a squeeze of lemon, and a pinch of Celtic salt. It's our mission this month to learn to appreciate the simplicity and learn to enjoy food the way it's meant to taste.

Dinner: Day 1

Keep it light tonight by serving your dinner on a smaller plate than you typically use. Remember to slow down, chew your food, focus on flavors and textures, and put your fork down in between bites. Food is meant to fuel your body but if we don't enjoy what we eat it can often lead to overdoing it. So get in touch with what your body is really craving, slow down and savor your meal!

Self Care

Today, I want you to get a massage. Whether it's a foot massage from your spouse, a quick massage at the mall, or a 60-minute deep tissue rub-down, focus on doing something to pamper your body and enhance your detoxification experience. Massages give you energy, improve circulation, boost your immune system, and improve sleep quality, so schedule some "you time" and get in the habit of making self-care a requirement!

Share with a friend the sticky note trick for getting your daily eight glasses of water! #liveitshareit

Day 2

Lemon Water And Cayenne

Yay! You did it! Your first day is over and you're one step closer to creating a healthy lifestyle you love.

Today, we're going to focus on one of my favorite simple steps to starting your day off right – warm lemon water. This is such an essential practice for your health but I'll try to keep it short and straightforward!

For starters, the practice stimulates the liver (the body's primary detoxifying organ) and energizes the digestive system. Your liver releases uric acid and creates bile to safely eliminate toxins. Keeping your liver and digestive system cleansed and in tip-top shape helps prevent chronic fatigue.

I love lemon juice and cayenne pepper for their anti-fungal and immune boosting properties. Lemon is a natural detoxifier as vitamin C transforms toxins into digestible material. In addition to vitamin C, lemons are also packed with antioxidants and electrolytes including potassium, calcium and magnesium. Lemon is also known to stimulate the liver's natural enzymes by helping to oxygenate the body and despite their acidity, lemons actually help neutralize the body's pH by making it more alkaline, aiding in weight loss. pH imbalance has been attributed to numerous disorders, including cancer.

Cayenne pepper in turn stimulates the circulatory system by opening the capillaries as well as aiding digestion and helping to regulate blood sugar. Furthermore, and very importantly, it increases the temperature of your body and kick-starts your metabolism.

After sleeping through the night, the bodily tissues are dehydrated and need clean, pure water to filter out toxins and improve energy production in the cells. Most individuals turn to stimulants like coffee in the morning to give them a jump-start. Unfortunately, coffee is a diuretic that depletes your body of water reserves and essential minerals and electrolytes like sodium, potassium, calcium and magnesium. Instead, by adding in lemon water, we're hydrating our cells resulting in an instant energy and mood boost. In fact, this lemon water boost can be so effective that you could even indulge in a little coffee afterwards and not have to worry about dehydration!

This beverage is best consumed first thing in the morning, on an empty stomach, BEFORE you brush your teeth (the buildup will help to protect your precious tooth enamel). I also recommend warming up your water just a bit and sipping through a straw. You can use as much or as little cayenne as you like but I typically add about one-eighth of a teaspoon in one quart of water with the juice of half a lemon. Cheers!

Here's Your Game Plan For Day 2!

Upon rising, start your day off with a mug of warm water with the juice of half a lemon and a small pinch of cayenne pepper. Sip that down followed by a cup of tea and then breakfast.

Do 50 jumping jacks. Ready set go!

Breakfast: Day 2

Craving comfort? Try my Green Power Bowl! It's loaded with protein and fiber to keep you full and energized all morning long. If you're running low on time in the mornings, try slicing up your greens, garlic, and onion ahead of time and just toss into the skillet as needed. Quinoa also works great in place of the rice if you're looking to switch things up a bit. Turn to page 122 for the recipe!

Lunch: Day 2

For lunch today, take last night's leftovers and pile them on top of a big bed of greens (it doesn't get much easier than that!). Use olive oil, lemon, and Celtic salt to dress, adding a little hummus, lentil dip, or baba ganoush if you want something with a bit more flavor.

Dinner: Day 2

Tonight, fix a delicious veggie soup such as butternut squash or kale and white bean for dinner. Sit and savor every bite as you nourish your body and relax!

Self Care

Today, I want you to focus on writing down and reciting three positive affirmations. Everything you think or say is an affirmation but negative thought patterns can cause subconscious sabotage as you pursue your goals.

You can use positive affirmations (which are usually short, positive statements) targeted at a specific set of beliefs to challenge and undermine negative feelings and to replace them with positive, self-nurturing thoughts.

To start your day, list three things you believe in, such as "I am healthy, I am beautiful, I deserve to love my body and life…" You get the picture. Write them on a sticky note or somewhere you will see them throughout the day and continue to remind yourself of how amazing you are.

I suggest doing this on a regular basis whenever you need encouragement or a pick-me-up!

Post a photo of your lemon water on Instagram. #liveitshareit

Green Power Bowl

1. Rinse rice and place in a rice cooker with water, flip the switch to cook and set aside. Alternatively, bring water to a boil, add rice, reduce heat and cook 20 minutes or until water is absorbed.

2. In the meantime, drizzle a little olive oil the bottom of a pan over medium/medium-high heat.

3. Cut kale into ribbons and slice the onion and garlic. Add kale garlic, and onions to the pan with a pinch of salt and red pepper flakes, tossing to coat. Cook until kale begins to look dry adding another drizzle of oil. Continue this process until kale is bright green and tender and onions are cooked through about 5-6 min.

4. Remove from the pan and add a little oil and crack each of the eggs. Cook for about two minutes with the yolk sunny side up and then flip to the other side and cook for another minute before removing the eggs from the pan.

Ingredients

1 cup Japanese rice

1½ cups water

1 bunch greens (kale, collards, Swiss chard, etc)

½ large red onion

1 tbsp olive oil

½ tsp Celtic salt

¼ tsp red pepper flakes

2 garlic cloves, sliced

4 eggs

Hot Sauce

5. To serve, layer rice followed by kale mixture, finishing with an egg. Drizzle with optional hot sauce and serve immediately. Serves four.

* If you're cooking for one, either cut the recipe down or divide leftover rice and greens into glass Tupperware and simply reheat by tossing into a skillet and then frying up the egg right before serving! Or you can pre-slice up greens, onion, and garlic and add to a skillet to cook as you need them!

Day 3

Bump Up Your Hydration

Our bodies need hydration for survival – in fact, water is even more essential than food. Every single cell, tissue, and organ in your body needs water to function properly and the more hydrated you are, the more efficiently everything operates. Over 60 percent of your body is made up of water and you use that water to maintain internal temperature, digest food, cleanse cells, and eliminate waste.

Unfortunately, most of us are chronically dehydrated which takes a toll on energy, mood, and health. As you become thirsty, your energy levels experience a serious drop. This tells your body to seek quick energy, often in the form of food with the most regular target being sugar. The problem here is that the energy drop is not because you're hungry but as a result of thirst, leading you to treat the symptom instead of the cause.

The great news, however, is that hydration is one of the simplest things you can do for your body and when done properly, it will have a tremendous impact on your long-term health. All it takes is eight glasses of pure, filtered water a day to boost energy, digestion, nutrient absorption, and eventually, weight loss!

For optimal hydration, I recommend drinking room temperature water if you can get used to it. When you drink ice-cold water, it causes your blood vessels to contract forcing your body to warm itself up by expending enzymes and energy needed for digestion.

Cold water is also less absorbent, which results in a slowing of the hydration process. Another simple way to bump up your hydration is to add water-dense foods such as cucumbers, watermelon, celery, apples, romaine lettuce, and citrus fruits into your daily lifestyle.

Here's Your Game Plan For Day 3!

Upon rising, start your day off with a mug of warm water with the juice of half a lemon and a small pinch of cayenne pepper. Sip that down followed by a cup of tea and then breakfast.

Add in some yoga. I love finding great 10-20 minute practices on YouTube that allow me to fit in some simple and quick stretching in the morning or evening.

Breakfast: Day 3

Overnight oats are the perfect breakfast for those mornings when you don't have a lot of time to spend in the kitchen, or just simply don't want to cook. Master the technique and then play around with whatever ingredients and mix-ins you like. Some of my favorites include cocoa powder, strawberries, almond or cashew butter, apples and cinnamon, hemp seeds, pumpkin butter, and cherries. Recipe page 129.

Lunch: Day 3

Savor your leftover soup with a side salad...or if you're feeling frisky, simply stir in some ribbons of spinach for a delicious one pot meal!

Dinner: Day3

Roasted vegetables are a staple in my refrigerator. They're amazing to keep on hand for quick snacks and to add to meals. Today, roast up some root veggies and serve them over some greens and quinoa, and top off with a delicious fried egg and a little hot sauce! Recipe page 130.

Self Care

Today, make an effort to laugh more. Laughter relaxes the whole body, boosts the immune system, decreases stress hormones and increases immune cells and infection-fighting antibodies, improving your resistance to disease.

Laughter also triggers the release of endorphins, the body's natural feel-good chemicals, which promote an overall sense of well-being. Regular giggling also protects the heart by improving the function of blood vessels and blood flow, which can help prevent heart attacks and other cardiovascular problems.

So today, focus on letting it all go and just laugh – you will feel amazing!

Bring an extra water bottle to the gym for your workout buddy. #liveitshareit

Oatmeal Raisin Cookie Overnight Oats

1. In a bowl, add the oats, chia seeds, cinnamon, and raisins. Whisk for five seconds or so until mixed. Add almond milk and whisk until the clumps are gone.

2. Place in fridge overnight or for two hours. In the morning, remove from fridge and drizzle with a bit of pure maple syrup and top with walnuts and banana slices.

Ingredients

¼ cup oats

½ cup non-dairy milk (I prefer almond milk)

½ tbsp chia seed

1 tbsp walnuts, chopped

¾ tsp cinnamon

½ tsp vanilla extract

1 tbsp raisins

½ banana, sliced (optional)

Maple syrup (optional)

Simple Roasted Root Vegetables

1. Preheat oven to 425 degrees.

2. Peel and cut carrots, parsnips and beets into even pieces.

3. Cut the stem off of each Brussels sprout, remove the outer layer and slice in half.

4. Quarter the onion and remove peels from the garlic cloves.

5. Add everything to a baking sheet, drizzle with oil and sprinkle with salt, red pepper, and herbs. Toss to coat and put it into the oven for 30-45 minutes until tender.

Ingredients

2 carrots

2 parsnips

2 beets

½lb Brussels sprouts

1 onion

4 garlic cloves

½ tsp Celtic salt

¼ tsp red pepper

2 tbsp olive oil

1 tsp herbs de Provence

Day 4

Cut Down The Caffeine

We know the importance of drinking plenty of water to stay hydrated but unfortunately, the drink of choice for most Americans is coffee. As much as we all love a good "cup of joe," this drug of choice does a number on our health.

Caffeine aggravates our nervous system, depletes us of many vitamins and minerals, and wreaks havoc on our adrenal glands. Although it is made with water, coffee actually dehydrates us and causes our bodies to become acidic. Too much caffeine can also affect sleep, cause anxiety or jitters, and weaken our bones, leading to osteoporosis down the road.

For the next 24 days, we're focusing on hydrating with plenty of water and herbal tea while saving coffee as a special treat. Instead of deprivation, simply focus on becoming aware, conscious, and mindful of your intake. Three cups of coffee a day is far too many – in fact for every caffeinated beverage consumed, you should plan to rehydrate with two glasses of water. The occasional unsweetened latte or cozy cup of coffee is perfectly fine as a Healthy Indulgence – just savor every sip and move on with your life.

If you think you can't possibly function without coffee, give it a few days. Once you get through your withdrawal, you'll realize you actually have more energy than you did when drinking coffee. If you need a little boost first thing in the morning, I recommend a cup of green tea. Green tea is naturally lower in caffeine than coffee, but is also great source of antioxidants and flavonoids, which protect our bodies from cancer causing free radicals.

Here's Your Game Plan For Day 4!

Upon rising, start your day off with a mug of warm water with the juice of half a lemon and a small pinch of cayenne pepper. Sip that down followed by a cup of tea and then breakfast.

Do 20 calf-raises while you brush your teeth in the morning and again at night!

Breakfast: Day 4

Raw fruits and veggies are extremely hydrating. Try this cucumber green smoothie as a nice alternative to some of the sweeter versions. Cucumbers are amazing for skin and hydration, and the healthy fats in the avocado will keep you full all morning long. Turn to page 135.

Lunch: Day 4

Make up this gorgeous Swiss chard and caramelized onion frittata and serve over a bed of mixed greens dressed with olive oil, lemon, and Celtic salt for a fabulous lunch! Turn to page 136.

Dinner: Day 4

Sauté some collard greens and serve with a piece of wild caught salmon!

Self Care

Take five minutes in the morning and just breathe. When you start your day in a relaxed rather than rushed state, you're more likely to make decisions that support your health.

Invite a friend over for a cup of herbal tea. Talk about your day. #liveitshareit

Cucumber Green Smoothie

1. Add ingredients to a blender and puree until smooth, adding more ice or water to reach desired consistency!

Ingredients

1 small cucumber (peeled if not organic)

¼ avocado

1 apple, cored

1 tbsp minced ginger

Juice of 1 lime

1 cup water

A few ice cubes

1 handful of spinach

Swiss Chard Caramelized Onion Frittata

1. In a medium bowl, beat eggs with two tablespoons of water and then add salt. Set aside. Heat olive oil in a medium skillet over medium heat and add the onion. At the same time, preheat the broiler.

2. Sauté the onion until it becomes a nice, golden color (about 10 minutes) and then add the chard and thyme to the pan. Cook until the chard wilts down and brightens in color.

Ingredients

2 tbsp extra virgin olive oil

6 leaves Swiss chard, cut into ribbons

1 small onion, sliced thinly

6 eggs

½ tsp Celtic salt

½ tsp fresh thyme

Freshly ground black pepper to taste

3. Spread evenly over the bottom of the pan and then pour in the egg mixture. Allow the mixture to set, pulling back the edges every now and then.

4. When the edges pull back easily from the pan and the center is only slightly runny, place it under the broiler for 5-10 minutes, until the top is lightly browned. Remove from oven and serve over a bed of mixed greens with a drizzle of olive oil and pinch of salt!

Day 5

Move Your Body

Today's focus is super important! In fact, it's so essential that it's actually one of my Six Habits of Healthy Living and an action that, when incorporated into your lifestyle, can transform your health. Your body is designed to move, but many of us spend the majority of the day sitting at a desk followed by a couch and then a bed with hardly any movement at all. On average, most Americans only squeeze in around 5,000 of the recommended 10,000+ steps we are supposed to take each day.

When you sit for an extended period of time, your body starts to shut down at the metabolic level. When muscles (especially the big ones meant for movement like those in your legs) are immobile, your circulation slows and you burn fewer calories. Key flab-burning enzymes responsible for breaking down triglycerides (a type of fat) simply start switching off. Sit for a full day and those fat burners plummet by as much as 50 percent.

And that's not all. The less you move, the less blood sugar your body uses. Research shows that for every two hours spent on your backside per day, your chance of contracting diabetes goes up by seven percent. Your risk for heart disease goes up too because enzymes that keep blood fats in check are inactive. You're also more prone to depression – with less blood flow, fewer feel-good hormones are circulating to your brain.

Think of your body as a computer – as long as you're moving the mouse and tapping the keys, all systems are on and running. But let it idle for a few minutes and the machine goes into power-conservation mode. Your body is meant to move, so when you sit and do nothing for too long, it shuts down and burns less energy. Getting steady activity throughout the day keeps your metabolism buzzing along in high gear.

The idea is that rather than obsessing over one 30-minute gym session per day, think of movement as a consistent objective. Make an effort to move your body first thing when you wake up (10 minutes on the rebounder or some quick yoga is my favorite), park a little further away at work, take the stairs, look for a further away restroom and walk for a few minutes at lunch.

After work, find some way to squeeze activity into your evening whether it's a long walk, gym time, some weight training, or yoga to unwind. Just a small shift in mindset from working out to simply moving your body can make all of the difference in the world.

Here's Your Game Plan For Day 5!

Upon rising, start your day off with a mug of warm water with the juice of half a lemon and a small pinch of cayenne pepper. Sip that down followed by a cup of tea and then breakfast.

Do 100 squats – I like to break this up into sets of 25 four times throughout the day. Watch your form and be sure to contract your abs to get the most out of this movement! Do your squats in the

bathroom, in your office, while you're on the phone – simply find the time and just do it!

Breakfast: Day 5

Grab your room temp frittata on the go or serve over greens for breakfast! Make sure to skip the microwave – it zaps the nutritional value of your food by as much as 97%. I like to reheat my foods in a skillet – once you get into the habit, you'll realize that it really doesn't take much time at all!

Lunch: Day 5

When I first started teaching cooking classes in college, my most popular class was "Healthy in a Hurry" and this soup was something I came back to again and again. It's seriously fool-proof, super fast and absolutely delicious! Turn to page 143.

Dinner: Day 5

Keep it simple and light tonight with some more soup and salad. Add a little cooked quinoa or millet to your salad and also a hard-boiled egg if you want a little more substance.

Self Care

Dry Brush! Daily dry brushing is a great way to get rid of dead skin cells while improving circulation and lightly stimulating your lymph system. Look for a natural bristle brush at your local health food store or online.

The best and most effective time to dry brush is before your shower or bath first thing in the morning. I start with my legs, brushing towards my heart, paying special attention to my legs and booty.

Remember to be kind – if it hurts a little at first, go gently (especially on your chest and neck) and your skin will get used to it. Make brushing part of your daily beauty regime and you'll find your skin will become super soft with the added bonus of an effortlessly boosted immune system.

Invite a friend to go for a walk. #liveitshareit

Creamy Black Bean Soup

1. Drain and rinse beans. Reserve ¼ cup and add the rest to your blender.

2. Add 1½ cups of vegetable stock, cumin, salsa, salt, and garlic and blend until smooth, adding more stock if needed. If using a Vitamix, blend 3-4 minutes or until hot. If using a regular blender, transfer mixture to a pot and warm over medium-low heat.

3. Stir in reserved beans, garnish with cilantro and drizzle with cashew crème (optional). Serves four.

Ingredients

2 cans black beans, drained and rinsed

1½ to 2 cups vegetable stock

⅓ cup prepared salsa (I like Trader Joe's Roasted Garlic)

½ tsp cumin

¼ tsp salt

1 clove garlic

Cilantro

Hot sauce (optional)

Cashew Crème

1. Add ¼ cup of cashews to a blender and cover with water, blending until smooth. Add the remaining cashews with the blender running until you reach a thick, cream-like consistency, adding water if needed. Drizzle cashew crème over prepared soup and serve!

Ingredients

½ cup cashews, soaked

Day 6

Rethink Exercise

Although moving your body is insanely important to your health, exercise should be fun. If dragging your butt to the gym every single day feels like a burden and stresses you out, it's probably causing more harm than good.

Here's the thing tension in the brain leads to tense habits. Eating for reward, emotional eating, and over-eating to "get through the tough workout" all come from tension in your mind and body. If you love your form of exercise, whether it's spinning, running, yoga, hiking, dancing, or whatever, that enjoyment is causing a reaction in your brain that will lead you in the direction of treating yourself well. Doing what you love leads to happiness and good health. The activity itself doesn't matter – what matters is how you feel about it.

The fabulous thing about my philosophy of creating a sustainable, long-term healthy lifestyle is that it's not about exercise but simply making an effort to move. Don't fixate on whether or the not you make it the gym six days a week – instead focus on making a conscious effort to move your body each and every day. I've found by doing this, exercise becomes fun and moving becomes habit. I also enjoy going to the gym a lot more the three or four days a week I do go rather than when I was forcing myself to go daily.

Consistency is key – if you can do it regularly and enjoy the process, it will be much easier to maintain!

Need inspiration? Try taking a long walk each evening after dinner to unwind; do a 30-minute yoga flow in the mornings to start your day off right; pick up a kettle bell and do 100 swings every few days to build muscle tone and get your heart rate up; look for fun DVDs you can do at home to keep things exciting; take a bike ride and pack a picnic for a fun way to get moving.

Exercise can be simple and a seamless addition to your lifestyle if you just get creative and start embracing daily movement.

Here's Your Game Plan For Day 6!

Upon rising, start your day off with a mug of warm water with the juice of half a lemon and a small pinch of cayenne pepper. Sip that down followed by a cup of tea and then breakfast.

Sit up straight! Sitting up straight instead of leaning back in the chair requires you to use the muscles in your back and in your abdominals and will also increase calorie burning while you're sitting at your desk. Good posture also helps you look slimmer and more youthful.

Breakfast: Day 6

Savory oats are a quick and simple breakfast. Cook steel cut or old fashioned oats in water and simply finish off with a drizzle of good extra virgin olive oil, a pinch of Celtic sea salt, and a few red pepper flakes or black pepper.

Lunch: Day 6

Top off some mixed greens with leftover roasted veggies and quinoa! If you haven't cooked quinoa before, I recommend picking up a rice cooker to simplify the process. Make sure to rinse your quinoa in a fine-mesh strainer to remove the outer coating and then simply use a 2:1 ratio of water to quinoa.

If you're cooking on the stovetop, I like to bring my water to a boil first and then cook for about 10 minutes until most of the water is absorbed. Then, I remove my pot from the heat and let sit another 5 minutes or so before serving.

Dinner: Day 6

Spaghetti squash is one of my favorites. Cut your squash in half, clean out the seeds and roast at 425 degrees until tender (about 45 minutes). Using a fork, create "noodles" and toss with a little olive oil, salt, and garlic. If you want to get fancy, top off with some burst tomato sauce and serve with arugula!

Self Care

Stop comparing yourself to others! When we focus on comparing our lives to those of others, we often dwell on the negative instead of the amazing things we have to be grateful for! Keep in mind, most people have their own struggles too but we just don't see them! So today focus on the only person you can control – you.

Tweet about how you are moving your body today! #liveitshareit

Day 7

Incorporate Yoga For Body Awareness

You're one week in and should be noticing a few small changes since you've started creating a healthier lifestyle. Congratulations on making it this far! Over the next week, we will continue to focus on small changes to create your long-term, sustainably healthy lifestyle. Today, we're talking mindfulness and yoga so let's get started.

The Yoga Sūtras of Patañjali defines yoga as "the stilling of the changing states of the mind". In a busy, over-stimulated world, it's so important to take the time to slow down and reconnect with the body and mind.

A yoga practice is the perfect medium to help increase awareness, allowing you to make better choices throughout the day as well as enhancing your enjoyment of life and overall happiness. Balancing exercises are also amazing for strengthening the physical body as well as calming and bolstering the nervous system.

The best part is that it doesn't have to take hours a day to practice yoga. I like to find free videos online or DVDs at the library and spend 15-20 minutes on my practice. If you have more time and want to spend a full hour, then go for it, but it doesn't take long to reap the benefits of yoga.

Also, don't forget to breathe. Connecting with your breath is one of the most important parts of yoga and is something most of us don't focus on enough, if at all. Concentrating on each inhalation and exhalation, while taking air deep into your lungs, allows tension to leave your body resulting in instant stress relief and a sense of balance.

Here's Your Game Plan For Day 7!

You know the drill – lemon H2O first and then breakfast!

Find a yoga class in town and take some time out of your day to connect your body and mind. Many studios offer the first class for free or at a discounted rate, so do a little research to find a good fit for your lifestyle.

Breakfast: Day 7

Scramble an egg or two and remove from the skillet. Drizzle half an avocado with olive oil and a pinch of Celtic salt and place face down in the same skillet. Cook until fragrant and lightly browned. To serve, fill seared avocado with eggs and top with arugula and hot sauce!

Lunch: Day 7

Make yourself a big ol' salad. Try adding some beans or cooked lentils for an extra nutritional boost!

Dinner: Day 7

Shred some Brussels sprouts and serve them over quinoa. Add a little meat or fish if you want it! Turn to page 155.

Self Care

Buy yourself fresh flowers! Simply buying yourself flowers is a great way of saying "I'm awesome! I deserve this." Take the time to bring a little beauty into your world. The smell of fresh flowers is calming and a great way to relieve stress. Don't wait till tomorrow; go buy yourself some flowers today.

You and a coworker go check out a new yoga studio. #liveitshareit

Shaved Brussels Sprouts

Ingredients

1 lb. Brussels sprouts

½ inch piece peeled ginger, sliced thin

4 cloves garlic, sliced

1 tbsp olive oil, divided.

¼ -½ tsp Celtic salt to taste

Pinch red pepper flakes

1. Halve Brussels sprouts and slice into thin ribbons, holding at the stem end. Set-aside and slice ginger and garlic.

2. Add a ½ tbsp olive oil in a skillet over medium heat with salt and red pepper. Cook for 4-5 minutes until Brussels sprouts are bright green and garlic and ginger are tender and fragrant, adding olive oil a drizzle at a time and tossing to coat. Finish with another light drizzle of oil and season to taste.

Day 8

Add In Weights

Now that you're moving your body daily, it's time to get a little more focused and add in some weight training. For me, weights are a perfect example of why I believe so strongly in the 80/20 Principle.

When you lift weights, you are not only boosting your metabolism in the short-term but for hours to follow. Minimal effort and time spent yields the maximum results – it's a no-brainer. Strength training not only boosts your metabolism and burns fat, but it's also important for increasing bone density, boosting stamina, sharpening your focus, and preventing chronic conditions like heart disease.

The best part is 2-3 days a week of weight training is all you really need to get results. Just keep in mind that it can be easy to injure yourself so if you're new to weight training, I suggest working with a professional to make sure you're building a strong foundation.

Here's Your Game Plan For Day 8!

Upon rising, start your day off with a mug of warm water with the juice of half a lemon and a small pinch of cayenne pepper. Sip that down followed by a cup of tea and then breakfast.

Always take the stairs no matter what. It's a simple way to squeeze in a little extra movement without even trying, plus stairs are great for toning your tush!

Breakfast: Day 8

Fix yourself some delish overnight oats! Switch up your toppings so you'll never get bored. Some of my favorites include; almond butter, walnuts, chia seeds, dried cherries, apple, dark chocolate, coconut butter, and dried coconut flakes.

Lunch: Day 8

Add some cauliflower into your life. It's amazing for cancer prevention as it supports your body's detox and anti-inflammatory systems, and is also a great source of antioxidants and vitamin C, which aid in boosting our immune system. Recipe page 160.

Dinner: Day 8

Make it predominately plant-based but add in a little extra protein such as a pan-roasted chicken thigh (or if you're vegetarian, try some beans)!

Self Care

Pick up tongue scraping. During sleep when the body is resting, the digestive system works to detoxify itself. These toxins are deposited on the surface of the tongue via the internal excretory channels and are responsible for the coating usually seen on the tongue first thing in the morning. Tongue scraping helps to gently detoxify your body each and every morning and is a great way to start your day off right!

Pin your favorite YouTube workout on Pinterest. #liveitshareit

Lemony Cauliflower And Fennel Soup

1. Preheat oven to 425 degrees. Place fennel and cauliflower flat on sheet pan and roast for 30 minutes, or until tender, turning occasionally. Remove from the oven and set aside.

2. Add olive oil to a large heavy bottomed pot over medium heat. Add the onions and sauté for 5 minutes, until translucent. Add the garlic and sauté for 1-2 minutes, until fragrant. Add the roasted fennel and cauliflower, vegetable stock, and beans. Bring to a boil and then simmer for 10-15 minutes. Stir in lemon juice and zest.

3. Blend the soup adding more liquid as needed.

Ingredients

1 large fennel bulb, chopped
1 large head cauliflower, chopped
1 tbsp olive oil
1 medium yellow onion, chopped
2 garlic cloves, sliced
4 cups vegetable stock or water + 1 vegetable stock cube
2 cups cooked white beans
Celtic salt
2 tbsp fresh parsley
2 organic lemons zest and juice
Olive oil for drizzling

Before serving, season with Celtic salt and black pepper to taste.

Garnish bowls with fresh parsley, lemon wedge and a drizzle of olive oil.

Day 9

Greens

Greens are at the foundation of a healthy lifestyle and are, in my opinion, one of the easiest ways to totally transform your health. Green leafy vegetables are an amazing source of vitamins, protein, minerals and fiber, and give us huge amounts of energy while filling us up at the same time. They help boost our immune system, are loaded with antioxidants to protect against disease, and are a simple way to provide balance to our meals as well as aiding in digestion and detoxification.

So here's the idea behind my approach. By consciously making an effort to add something green to each meal, you're able to effortlessly bump up the nutrient density of your plate. You're filling up on less, boosting energy, feeling better, and gently detoxifying your body daily.

Most importantly, becoming more conscious about your health and taking small steps each day will result in instant gratification and desire to continue on this path. When you feel good, you don't need motivation to sustain a healthy lifestyle in the long term – you just need simple, practical solutions you can implement daily and bumping up your intake of greens is just one such solution.

Here's how I get my greens in daily.

Breakfast: Start your day off with a green smoothie or juice; throw a fried egg on a bed of greens; stir sautéed greens into a frittata and then serve with some spinach; wrap up your favorite breakfast burrito ingredients in romaine or collards; build a power breakfast bowl with sautéed greens, quinoa or rice, and a fried, poached, or hardboiled egg on top or; cook oatmeal and garnish with thinly sliced spinach, olive oil, salt and red pepper.

Lunch: Serve last night's leftovers over a big salad; stir greens into hot soup to wilt; make wraps with collards or romaine and your favorite fillings (hummus, sweet potatoes, black beans, egg salad, tuna salad, chickpea salad…) or; massage some kale.

Dinner: Add some sautéed greens in with your meal; serve your meal over spinach, arugula, or mixed greens; thinly slice and sauté

Brussels sprouts; top your meal off with some baked kale chips or; stir thinly sliced nori into warm rice. With a little creativity, the possibilities are endless!

Here's Your Game Plan For Day 9!

Don't forget to start your day off right with your new favorite spicy and citrus beverage before breakfast!

Use TV commercials as an exercise break while you're watching your favorite shows. Plan ahead of time to do jumping jacks during the first break, crunches during the second, and squats during the third. It's an easy way to squeeze in a little extra movement while indulging

in some TV time!

Breakfast: Day 9

Try some chia pudding! Chia seeds are a great food to include into your new healthy lifestyle. They're a great source of omega 3 fats, which are important for brain health and are also loaded with fiber, an essential for digestion and weight loss. Turn to page 168.

Lunch: Day 9

Massaging your kale is in order today and if this is the first time you've ever had raw kale, you're in for an enzyme-rich treat! Turn to page 171.

Dinner: Day 9

Make your favorite dinner and serve it over a bed of greens (mixed greens, spinach, arugula, baby kale…whichever you prefer!)

Self Care

Go to sleep 30 minutes earlier tonight, Sleep has a huge impact on your immune function as well as how your body processes blood glucose.

To get the most benefit from your sleep plan, try to get to bed at least 15 minutes earlier each night and create a pre-bedtime routine to help you unwind. Take a warm bath, light some incense, read a book, turn on some peaceful music, or spritz your pillow with essential oil. Also keep electronic use to a minimum 30 minutes before bed.

So unplug, kick back and prepare yourself for a fabulous night sleep!

Make a green smoothie for your favorite morning buddy!
#liveitshareit

Pumpkin Chia Pudding

1. Combine all of the ingredients in a blender and blend until a uniform texture is achieved.

2. Transfer to a sealed container and allow to chill overnight.

** store bought almond milk is a good option but if you have the time, I HIGHLY suggest making your own at home in about 5 minutes.

** Alternatively, you can whisk ingredients together if you don't want to blend.

Ingredients

3 tbsp chia seeds

1 cup almond milk**

1 tsp vanilla extract

1 tbsp pure maple syrup or one date

¼ cup canned pumpkin

1 tsp pumpkin pie spice

Almond Milk

1. Soak the almonds overnight or up to two days**. Place the almonds in a bowl and cover with about an inch of water. They will plump as they absorb water. Let stand, uncovered, overnight or up to two days. The longer the almonds soak, the creamier the almond milk.

Ingredients

1 cup raw almonds, preferably organic

2 cups water, plus more for soaking

Sweeteners – dates, maple syrup, stevia (optional)

Vanilla extract (optional)

2. Drain and rinse the almonds. Combine the almonds and water in a blender. Place the almonds in the blender and cover with two cups of water. Blend at the highest speed for two minutes. Pulse the blender a few times to break up the almonds and then blend continuously for two minutes. The almonds should be broken down into a very fine meal and the water should be white and opaque. (If using a food processor, process for four minutes total, pausing to scrape down the sides halfway through.)

3. Strain mixture through a nut milk bag or cheesecloth, squeeze and press with clean hands to extract as much almond milk as possible. You should get about two cups. Sweeten to taste and keep

refrigerated for up to three days.

** Soaking the almonds is not only an essential step for creamy, delicious milk but is also super important to increase the digestibility and nutrient assimilation of the almonds. I recommend getting in the habit of soaking all of your almonds for at least a few hours before consuming. You can do a few cups at a time and keep them stored in the refrigerator. You'll get more out of your almonds and ease your digestion.

Massaged Kale Salad

1. In a large serving bowl, add the kale, half of the lemon juice, a drizzle of oil and a little kosher salt. Massage for about 2-3 minutes or until the kale starts to soften and wilt. Set aside while you make the dressing.

2. In a small bowl, whisk remaining lemon juice with the honey and lots of freshly ground black pepper. Stream in the oil while whisking until a dressing forms, and you like how it tastes. Pour the dressing over the kale and add the apple, cranberries, and walnuts. Toss and serve.

Ingredients

1 bunch kale, stalks removed and discarded, leaves thinly sliced

1 small lemon, juiced

2-3 tbsp extra-virgin olive oil, plus extra for drizzling

Celtic salt

2 tsp honey

Freshly ground black pepper

1 small granny smith apple, diced

¼ cup walnuts, toasted

2 tbsp cranberries, dried

Day 10

Change Up Your Plate

Today's the day to forget everything you have ever learned about square meals and the food pyramid. Instead, we're shifting our focus to rethinking what goes onto our plate. So far, I have been emphasizing the importance of a plant-based diet and filling your plate with greens, but now it's time to dive a little deeper into the reasoning behind my philosophy and exactly why it works.

The idea behind a plant-based diet isn't to say that you should never have meat. However, with plants being the most nutrient-dense foods on the planet, doesn't it make sense to make them the cornerstone of our diet?

From a weight-loss perspective, plant-based foods are naturally low in calories and high in nutrients and fiber, causing you to fill up and get all of the nutrition your body needs while simply eating less.

Plants also give us energy and make us feel good, two essentials for living a healthy lifestyle. And when we feel good, we are better able to sustain our lifestyle in the long term! Whenever we have a bad day, we recognize how good we feel with our healthier habits and actually look forward to getting back on track, no motivation or willpower required.

So here's the deal. Making plants the foundation of your diet takes some practice, but like anything else, once you get in the habit it becomes second nature. I always shoot for 60-75 percent of my plate to be filled with vegetables and then the rest can be whatever I like. For example, when I build my plate, I start with some sort of green (raw or cooked) such as sautéed kale and then add another vegetable, like acorn squash stuffed with quinoa, walnuts, celery, carrots, mushrooms, and fresh herbs.

Another example might be some raw spinach topped off with Japanese rice, a sweet potato, and fried egg – super simplistic but full of flavor and fiber. When you begin eating this way regularly, your blood sugar becomes naturally balanced, putting you in control of your cravings and increasing your awareness of what your body actually needs.

Here's Your Game Plan For Day 10!

Upon rising, start your day off with...well, you know!

Make an effort today to take 10 minutes and go for a walk either before or after your meals. As soon as you get up in the morning, take a quick stroll around the block; go for a walk at work during your lunch break; take 10 minutes in the evening to unwind and aid in digestion post-meal by taking a short walk. It's amazing how the little things add up, so do what

you can each day. Every little bit helps!

Breakfast: Day 10

This smoothie is loaded with iron and magnesium to give you plenty of energy all morning long. I love it simply because chocolate for breakfast makes me feel totally indulgent, even if it is a Healthy Indulgence! Turn to page 177.

Lunch: Day 10

Throw together a salad with whatever you've got in the refrigerator and top it off with some hummus and gluten/dairy free crackers (I recommend Mary's).

Dinner: Day 10

If you take the time to roast your sweet potatoes ahead of time, this soup comes together in just a few minutes, making this the perfect comfort meal for those busy weeknights! Turn to page 178.

Self Care

Put on a little makeup. How we look has a MAJOR impact on how we feel about ourselves and it is so often overlooked. Today, I want you to make an effort to do your hair, put on makeup, and slip on a nice outfit that you feel good in. Whether you are leaving the house or not, you'll feel sexy, confident, and will probably nourish your body a little better. When you feel good about yourself, you naturally make better choices and take care of your beautiful body!

Post a photo of your amazing dinner on Instagram. #liveitshareit

Chocolate Cherry Smoothie

1. Add ingredients to a blender and blend until smooth, adding ice/liquid as needed!

Ingredients

2 handfuls of fresh spinach

1½ cups almond milk

1 cup frozen cherries

1 banana, frozen

¼ avocado

2 tbsp raw cacao powder

Pinch of cinnamon

Ice

African-Inspired Sweet Potato Soup

1. Wrap the sweet potatoes in foil and roast until tender (425 degrees for about 45 minutes).

2. Add roughly chopped onions to a pot over medium heat with 1 tbsp coconut oil and salt. Sauté until soft (about six minutes), add in garlic and ginger and cook another 2-3 minutes.

3. Add in cooked sweet potatoes (skin optional – I leave it on) with berbere, vegetable stock cube, peanut butter, and enough water to combine.

Ingredients

3-4 sweet potatoes

½ red onion

3 cloves garlic

1 tsp minced ginger

1 tbsp coconut oil

1¼ tsp Celtic salt

1½ tbsp berbere

1 vegetable stock cube

2 tbsp organic peanut butter

Water

Spinach

Peanuts

4. Pour mixture into a blender and blend until smooth adding water until desired consistency is reached. Taste and adjust seasonings. To serve, top with spinach cut into ribbons and chopped, toasted peanuts!

Day 11

Balance Blood Sugar

Your blood sugar level is the amount of glucose circulating in your bloodstream gained from the food you've eaten and it's used to provide energy to cells immediately or be stored for future use. A well-balanced blood sugar level is essential to your overall health and well-being, as well as regulating hormones, triggering your body to burn stored fat, and increasing your metabolism to help you lose weight.

Unfortunately, most people's blood sugar is not properly balanced. When you consume too much glucose, it leads to high blood-sugar levels, causing your body to store excess as fat. Eating too little glucose can lead to a low blood sugar level, causing your body to go into "starvation mode" where it burns lean muscle instead of the fat.

Filling up on fiber-rich, plant-based foods is an essential part of keeping your blood sugar balanced, reducing the likelihood of mood swings. Today, we're going to focus on limiting your sugar intake and including plenty of greens and healthy fats such as olive oil, avocado and nuts with each meal to help keep that blood sugar in balance.

Want to take it a step further? Try bumping up your cinnamon intake. Just half a teaspoon per day helps regulate blood sugar by slowing the emptying of our stomach to reduce the sharp rise in blood sugar following meals. Cinnamon also plays a role in improving the effectiveness and sensitivity of insulin. I like to get a little cinnamon in each day by adding half a teaspoon to a large glass of water with one teaspoon of raw apple cider vinegar or by sprinkling a few pinches over sliced apples with some almond butter for dipping!

Here's Your Game Plan For Day 11!

Lemon? Check! Cayenne Pepper? Check! Time for breakfast!

Go for a bike ride. It's a fun way to get in touch with your inner child and fit in some great exercise. Try packing a picnic lunch for an even more special experience.

Breakfast: Day 11

Sauté some plantains in a little coconut oil and serve over mixed greens with a fried egg. Make a conscious effort today to add a little fat (avocado, olive or coconut oil , nuts) in with each meal to keep everything in balance. Plus, don't forget those fiber-rich greens!

Lunch: Day 11

Serve a homemade or prepared (check the ingredients) veggie burger over a bed of mixed greens with hummus, avocado, and lots of veggies. Add some probiotic rich sauerkraut or kimchi for an additional healthy boost.

Dinner: Day 11

Roast up some spaghetti squash and serve with tomato sauce, (made by simply adding cherry tomatoes, garlic, salt, olive oil, and herbs to a skillet and cooking until tomatoes burst) white beans, and sautéed kale.

A touch of goat cheese is also a great addition if you're looking for a Healthy Indulgence. Although I am not a huge fan of dairy, I do prefer using a small amount of delicious, grass-fed organic butter over margarine any day and occasionally I do indulge in some goat dairy.

Goat and sheep milk are much easier on our digestive systems because unlike cow dairy, milk enzymes are still present in goat and sheep dairy after pasteurization. So when going for dairy remember to make it an experience and enjoy every bite.

Self Care

Spend some time pampering yourself today. Try this simple face mask! Combine half a cup of hot – not boiling – water and a third of a cup of oatmeal. After a few minutes, stir in two tablespoons of plain yogurt, two tablespoons of honey, and an egg white. Apply to face and let sit for 10-15 minutes. Rinse with warm water!

Tell a loved one about the health benefits of coconut oil. #liveitshareit

Day 12

Focus On Raw

Raw foods are absolutely amazing for us but I find a lot of people begin cooking and forget to simply enjoy foods in their raw state as well. The number one reason why live foods are so important in our diet is a little something known as enzymes.

Enzymes, by definition, are large biological molecules that are responsible for thousands of metabolic processes that sustain life. Most importantly, they're responsible for aiding in the digestion of the food we consume. Research on enzymes has shown the importance of including raw foods in our diet to support healthy digestion and absorption of nutrients. These raw-food enzymes start the process of digestion in the mouth and upper stomach but when food is heated beyond 118 degrees, the enzymes are deactivated. Our bodies do produce their own enzymes for digestion but it helps when we get them from our foods as well.

Now this doesn't mean I am advocating a high-raw vegan diet (some foods are actually more nutritious when cooked), but the idea is to create the awareness that balance is key. Try to add raw fruits and veggies to your meals whenever you can (especially during the warmer months). Plus, raw foods are often a breeze to prepare (how easy is it to throw a handful of spinach on top of some soup?)! So cultivate your awareness, absorb more nutrients, improve digestion, and add a little more "raw" into your life.

Here's Your Game Plan For Day 12!

Don't forget to hydrate first thing when you wake up!

Find a set of hand weights either at home or at the gym and do 3 sets of 12 bicep curls.

Breakfast: Day 12

Like my overnight oats, this buckwheat parfait is one of those dishes you can switch up based on what you enjoy or have on hand. Try sweetening with honey, maple syrup, or dates and layer with fruit and nuts in a parfait dish to make breakfast a little more special! Turn to page 189.

Lunch: Day 12

Spring rolls are a great way to squeeze in a ton of raw vegetables. Make them super-satisfying by dipping them in a delicious peanut or almond butter sauce!

Dinner: Day 12

Serve dinner over a big bed of leafy greens! It's best to keep portions in check in the evening to ease digestion and allow your body to spend time on repair while you sleep. Also, try to eat at least three hours before you go to sleep.

Self Care

Eat without distractions! It's super-important to sit down and focus on exactly what is going into your mouth. Don't eat and read a magazine, watch TV, or check email at the same time. Multi-tasking is detrimental to most aspects of our life, especially when eating. Focusing on eating without distractions ensures that we eat just enough, burn more calories, have optimal digestion and most importantly, actually enjoy and taste our food.

So today, focus on the event of eating. Chew each bite, taste the flavors and appreciate the textures of your food. Eating should be a pleasurable experience and when you become better in tune with enjoying your meals, you'll recognize when you've had enough. Do this every time you put something in your mouth – no excuses!

Massage some kale and share a salad for lunch. #liveitshareit

Raw Buckwheat Breakfast Parfait

1. Soak the buckwheat overnight in two cups of filtered water.

2. The next morning, drain, rinse and pour into a food processor with almond milk. Process until smooth, adding in cinnamon, chia, stevia, and a pinch of salt.

3. Layer with optional mix-ins such as fresh fruit and raw nuts. Serves two.

Ingredients

½ cup buckwheat, soaked overnight and rinsed

¼ cup homemade almond milk

1 tbsp chia

1 tbsp maple syrup or stevia to taste

½ tsp cinnamon

1 tsp vanilla extract

Optional mix ins:

Hemp seeds (healthy balance of omega 3s and 6s)

Cashews (choose raw for optimal healthy fats)

Banana

Raisins

Strawberries (loaded with immune boosting vitamin C)

Day 13

Write It Down

It's simple – writing cultivates awareness. Whether it be scheduling workouts, keeping a food diary, or menu planning, things become real when we write them down.

Today, I want you to make a conscious effort to track everything you do from what goes into your mouth (even if it's just a bite) to how you move your body (squats, walks, jumping jacks, gym time, etc.) to how we feel before and after our meals, as well as any emotions that may cause us to eat.

Writing down food intake helps in a variety of ways but it also plays on your mind as you're less likely to eat something that you don't really want when you know that you have to write it down!

Food diaries also help you to become aware of habits such as snacking, emotional eating, or overdoing the sweets that you otherwise may not realize. They also help you to recognize gaps in your dietary intake, such as a lack of veggies, greens, or variety. Lastly, most of us don't get enough water, so keeping track really helps make that goal a reality!

I'm also a fan of penciling in workouts. Spend some time on Sundays looking over your week and try to figure out when you can make it to the gym, take a yoga class, go for a walk, or just spend time being active. I also love to do this with cooking. I often prep ahead for those weeknights when I know that I'll be busy or cook a larger quantity of soup or quinoa salad to have on hand for the week.

Bottom line – start recording and writing down anything that will help you better establish and stick to your healthy lifestyle.

Here's Your Game Plan For Day 13!

I think some lemon and cayenne water would be just the thing before my tasty (and healthy!) breakfast.

Spend time in the kitchen instead of on the couch. You may think you're too tired to cook at first, but once you start moving and cooking, you'll get an energy boost. Plus, by preparing and eating healthier meals, you'll naturally have more energy and won't need as much time to relax on the couch.

Breakfast: Day 13

Cook some oatmeal and serve with a drizzle of olive oil, a pinch of Celtic salt, red pepper, and thinly sliced spinach.

Lunch: Day 13

Fix a big, green salad and top with some cooked quinoa, tempeh, and roasted root veggies. Finish off with some olive oil, lemon, and Celtic salt.

Dinner: Day 13

This soup is another one that is super simple to prepare while also being ultra-rich and creamy. Try swapping out the vegetable stock for some coconut milk to change things up a bit. And if you're into dirtying one less dish, simply toss your onion and garlic on the sheet pan with diced squash and roast everything together! Just keep an eye on everything, as it will cook a little quicker. Turn to page 195.

Self Care

Watch the sunset! The sun sets every day and it's the most beautiful sight, but we rarely take the time to enjoy it. Go by yourself or with someone you care about and just sit in silence and enjoy the moment. This small act can totally transform your day and create an overwhelming sense of gratitude for your amazing life.

Write your workout plans on a sticky note and post a pic of it on Instagram. Instant accountability! #liveitshareit

Curried Butternut Squash Soup

Ingredients

1 large butternut squash (about 4 lbs)

1 vegetable stock cube

2-3 cups of water

2 tbsp curry

1 small yellow onion, diced

2 cloves of garlic, sliced

¼ tsp Celtic salt

Olive oil to garnish

1. Preheat oven to 425 degrees. Halve squash, scoop out seeds and place on a baking sheet. Drizzle with oil and sprinkle with salt. Bake for about 45 minutes until tender, flipping halfway through.

2. In the meantime, sauté the onion in ½ tbsp of olive oil until tender.

3. Stir in garlic and remove from heat.

4. Once squash has cooled enough to handle, scoop out flesh and add to pot with onion and garlic. Stir in vegetable stock cube and curry.

5. Puree mixture in a blender, adding water until desired consistency is reached. Drizzle with a touch of olive oil and a pinch of salt right before serving.

Day 14

Spend Time Planning Meals

Woohoo! We're two weeks in today and should be feeling fantastic. This healthy lifestyle thing ought to be starting to get a little easier and healthy choices are now becoming habit. Hopefully at this point you're also starting to have a little fun! Today we're going to focus on taking some time to plan so when things get a little crazy, you have healthy options to get you through.

Let's be honest, when your schedule is busy, the worst thing you can do is fuel your body with crap. Nutrient-lacking foods drain our energy and immune system and when we're busy, we simply don't have time to be sick and tired.

My solution is simple. Take a little time at the beginning of each week to look over your schedule and plan when you can cook and when you'll need to just grab and go. Then, figure out a few dishes to make for the week that you know will yield leftovers such as a pot of soup, roasted chicken and veggies, or a quinoa salad.

When you do your shopping, pick up the ingredients you need to make your staple dishes plus a little extra of whatever looks good that day. This method gives you the ability to know what you're having for dinner on those nights when you're feeling not-so-creative but also allows for leftovers on the days when you're simply too busy to cook. Plus, stocking your home with plenty of fresh produce means that when you do have a little time, you can whip up something fabulous!

I also recommend creating a list of staples to keep on hand so you always have something healthy to grab. For me some of those include: eggs, Japanese rice, seaweed snacks, mixed greens, spinach, hummus, Mary's crackers, apples, raw almond or organic peanut butter, quinoa and raw nuts. Stock up on those staples that work for you so that healthy and delicious food can be ready quicker than a trip to the drive-thru!

Here's Your Game Plan For Day 14!

Upon rising, start your day off with a mug of warm water with the juice of half a lemon and a small pinch of cayenne pepper. Sip that down followed by a cup of tea and then breakfast. I hope you didn't forget!

Try a rebounder. They're inexpensive and a lot of fun. Jumping up and down on a trampoline improves lymph system circulation, which in turn stimulates the immune system.

Breakfast: Day 14

Serve up a green smoothie this morning. Turn to page 201.

Lunch: Day 14

Leftover soup and a salad dressed with a little olive oil, Celtic salt, and lemon juice.

Dinner: Day 14

Try something new! Whether it's a new fruit or veggie, grain, meat or fish, make an effort tonight to pick out a new recipe and cook! Don't forget to make time to sit down and savor each bite and, of course, add a little something green!

Self Care

Get a pedicure! As one of my favorite self-care actions, pedis are an affordable luxury and make you feel like a million bucks when you leave the salon. Whether it's summertime or the middle of winter, indulge in a nice pedicure to get all that extra skin off your heels and unveil sexy feet you can be proud of. If no one will even see your feet, it's even more of an excuse to choose a wild color so schedule an appointment and pamper those feet!

Share some of your favorite recipes on a Pinterest Board called Healthy Living Redefined ;) #liveitshareit

Pineapple Mango Green Smoothie

1. Combine all of the ingredients in a blender. Blend until smooth and serve. Makes one large smoothie.

Ingredients

1 cup almond milk

½ banana, frozen

½ cup chopped mango

½ cup chopped fresh pineapple

2 cups fresh spinach

½ cup of ice

Day 15

Find Some Accountability

No matter where you're at in your lifestyle transition, accountability is key. I find that those who follow my philosophy of "Live It. Share It" have much higher rates of long-term success than those who keep their healthy lifestyle to themselves.

If you're in it for the long haul, doesn't it make sense to let everyone know what you're up to? This not only gives you a sense of accomplishment as you make changes, but also holds you accountable for those days when you're a little less than motivated.

When you have a friend to cook delicious, healthy food or go for a long walk with, things become that little bit more fun (aka easy to stick to). That's what this lifestyle is all about. I believe that the best way to learn is to teach, so it's time to start sharing your new lifestyle with everyone you know!

Surrounding yourself with like-minded people helps you stay committed as well as building you up! If you haven't yet, make sure to join my online community and use the hash tag *#liveitshareit* to connect with like-minded friends!

Here's Your Game Plan For Day 15!

Make sure to start your day off right and set yourself up for success!

Schedule exercise into your week. Sit down, look at your calendar and make it happen.

Breakfast: Day 15

Cook some oatmeal with an apple, dried cranberries, fresh cinnamon, and a little coconut.

Lunch: Day 15

Include lentils. They're naturally low in carbohydrates, high in protein and fiber, and a delicious addition to a salad or over some rice with greens. Plus, they can be stored in the fridge for up to five days so cook a few extra to grab throughout the week.

Dinner: Day 15

Roast up a big batch of seasonal veggies (recipe on page 130) using whatever seasoning and vegetables you like and serve over greens with chicken, tempeh, beans, or fish.

Self Care

Today, I want you to take some time and cook a nice dinner for yourself. So often we rush around the

kitchen to get food on the table fast — which is fine —
but on occasion, it's good to take some time to plan a
nice dinner, spend an hour or two shopping and
cooking, and sit down to a nicely set table with
candles and linens. Make dinner an experience, eat
slowly and share with someone special!

Tell a friend your goals and desires for a healthy lifestyle. #liveitshareit

Day 16

Keep A Food Diary:
Here's How

On Day 13, we covered the importance of writing things down and briefly discussed why I believe food diaries are crucial for creating a sustainably healthy lifestyle. At this point in my journey, I rarely write down my food intake and instead focus on recording my exercise and workouts, with the occasional bit of menu planning.

However, back when I was struggling with my own diet, I often relied on food diaries to get me back on track. The idea behind recording your intake is to cultivate awareness and point out areas that can be improved upon. We're often so busy that we go through our days mindlessly putting things in our mouth without really thinking about what we're actually consuming. When we write things down, we're better able to pinpoint where improvements can be made to get back on track.

When I keep a diary, I record the following: what I eat; when I eat it; how much (not in calorie count or specific measurements but in number of portions, taking one portion to be equal to a medium apple in size); where I am eating (on the couch, in the car, at the table); thoughts that are occurring as I am eating (as well as after); emotions (such as stress, relaxation, etc) and finally; saticty (am I full, stuffed, still a little hungry).

All of these details allow me to understand what is going on and where I can improve. Also, if I notice that I'm eating in the car or in front of the computer a little too often, I can tweak my schedule to allow more time to focus on what I am eating instead of shoving food into my mouth on the run.

What we eat is essential in reaching a healthy lifestyle but getting enjoyment and pleasure out of your food is will let you enjoy life and have a body you love. So spend the next week getting really clear on what's going into your body and why, so you can create the habits necessary to nourish your body long-term.

And to help you out, here is an example of what my food diary for a day might look like now.

7 a.m: Lemon water, 1.5 portions of white Japanese rice, one portion arugula and one egg. Eaten at the kitchen table, hungry but thoroughly enjoying the warmth and comfort of breakfast. I'm focused on what I am eating and satisfied as I finish. I sip on a cup of green tea and two glasses of water throughout the morning.

10 a.m: Post-workout green smoothie sipped at my desk with ½ a banana, a few blueberries, one scoop protein powder, four cups of spinach, water, 1 tsp maca, 1 tbsp chia seeds, ¼ avocado, and ice. I am enjoying the creamy texture of the smoothie and am satisfied as I finish.

1 p.m: A little hungry. I throw together four portions of mixed greens and top off with two portions of roasted veggies and ½ portion of cooked white beans. I finish off with a drizzle of olive oil, Celtic salt, and some lemon. I also have one portion of crackers on the side. I crave the crunch of the crackers which I find really satisfy me and enjoy all of the flavors and textures in the salad. I want something a little sweet so I brew a cup of herbal tea and sip on two glasses of water with lemon and apple cider vinegar throughout the afternoon.

6 p.m: *By this time I am hungry. I focus on only eating enough to be satisfied as I want to give my body time to digest my meal before bed. Often dinnertime is the most indulgent meal for me, but* *also the smallest portion as I enjoy a glass of wine and piece of dark chocolate on most nights.* Tonight I fixed one portion of fresh pasta tossed in olive oil and garlic with one portion of arugula and a few sun-dried tomatoes. This meal was definitely a Healthy Indulgence for me. I also sip on one glass of water after dinner. I feel satisfied after dinner, definitely not stuffed and very relaxed.

Here's Your Game Plan For Day 16!

Upon rising, start your day off with the hydrating goodness of warm lemon water followed by a cup of tea and then breakfast.

Grab a pedometer and track your steps. Make an effort to beat the day before and reward yourself with a new fitness top or cute new shoes when you reach your goals. Remember to take

things one day at a time and make it your goal to simply do better than you did the day before.

Breakfast: Day 16

Sometimes there's nothing better on a weekend than pancakes for breakfast. I use oats in this recipe to add extra fiber for blood sugar balance. If you enjoy maple syrup with your pancakes, go for the good stuff (local if possible) and remember, a little bit goes a long way! Turn to page 212.

Lunch: Day 16

Use those leftover roasted vegetables to make a vegetable and quinoa salad and serve over mixed greens. To switch things up a bit, dress your salad with some white balsamic or apple cider vinegar.

Dinner: Day 16

Roast a whole chicken with lots of veggies. If you're a

vegetarian just do the veggies, serve over some quinoa or millet with lentils and top with a fried egg.

Self Care

Take a bath! There's nothing better than taking half an hour out of your day to lounge in the tub. Make it special by lighting some candles, indulging in some fancy organic bath salts, and savoring the quiet! You deserve the downtime.

Share your food diary with your health coach. #liveitshareit

Pumpkin Oat Pancakes

1. Whisk together pumpkin puree, almond milk, eggs, coconut oil, maple syrup, vanilla bean paste, and orange juice. Stir in oat flour, salt, baking powder, cinnamon, and nutmeg.

2. Drop batter by spoonfuls into pre-heated skillet over medium heat with a little coconut oil to prevent sticking and cook 2-3 minutes per side until pancakes are cooked through. Serve with cinnamon and a little maple syrup!

Ingredients

1 cup oat flour

¾ cup pumpkin puree

½ tsp Celtic salt

¾ tsp baking powder

2 tbsp almond milk

½ orange juiced (or about 2-3 tbsp orange juice)

1 tsp cinnamon

½ tsp nutmeg

2 eggs

1½ tbsp coconut oil

1 tsp maple syrup

1 tsp vanilla bean paste

Day 17

Variety Is Key

So many people create a healthy lifestyle around eliminating certain foods but never incorporate new ones. I've even noticed some finding what works for weight loss for a short period of time, even if it means eating the same 5-6 foods over and over again. While those approaches may work for some people, they're simply not sustainable in the long term and are certainly not enjoyable.

Variety is key in the diet for two reasons. From a health perspective, our bodies need a variety of vitamins, minerals, and nutrients. Even with a whole-food, plant-based diet, without variety we're not able to get everything we need so it's important to include a wide selection of "colors" on your plate each day.

From a lifestyle perspective, variety is essential to help create a long-term, sustainably healthy lifestyle. When we eat the same things over and over again, eventually we get bored and overdo it in one way or another.

So think of variety as the spice of life and make trying new things into a fun challenge. Hit the local co-op, farmers market, or health food store and pick out one or two new things each week to incorporate into your life. It will keep things exciting and you might realize you love things you never knew existed! Exchange recipes with friends or spend some time looking for inspiration on blogs, Foodgawker, Pinterest, and in cookbooks/magazines.

Here's Your Game Plan For Day 17!

Mmmmm…warm lemon water. What a great way to kick off the day before eating breakfast!

Rent a new workout DVD from the library and complete one workout at

home!

Breakfast: Day 17

Get your green on with this anti-oxidant-rich, cancer-fighting smoothie! Turn to page 217.

Lunch: Day 17

Throw some raw veggies, sauerkraut, cooked rice, and sardines over mixed greens and dress with a little olive oil, lemon and Celtic salt.

Dinner: Day 17

I love serving tacos and burritos in greens. It's a fun way to lighten up your entire meal and keep everything fresh. Since making this swap, I find I actually really enjoy the crunch of the lettuce wrapping up my taco. The filling can easily be made up ahead of time and reheated in a skillet as needed. Also, feel free to add some grass-fed ground beef in with your tacos if you like. Turn to page 218.

Self Care

Sit down with a glass of wine (or tea) and piece of dark chocolate. Really pay attention to the flavors, textures, smells and tastes you're experiencing. And make sure when indulging to buy the best you can afford! You deserve it.

Bring a friend to the local farmer's market. Buy a vegetable you've never tried before! #liveitshareit

Strawberry And Green Tea Smoothie

1. Add all of the ingredients into a blender and blend until smooth adding ice or water as needed. Serve immediately.

Ingredients

6 fresh or frozen organic strawberries

1 cup washed baby spinach

½ cup frozen banana

½ cup almond milk

1 tbsp chia seed

½ cup fresh brewed unsweetened green tea

Sweet Potato And Black Bean Burritos

1. Preheat oven to 400 degrees. Peel and dice sweet potatoes and place on a lined baking sheet. Drizzle with olive oil and sprinkle with salt. Bake for 30 minutes until browned, turning once.

2. In the meantime, heat 1 tbsp olive oil in a large pan over medium heat. Add diced onion and ½ tsp salt and sauté until tender (around 5 minutes).

3. Stir in garlic and cook a few minutes before adding in cumin, chili powder, and lime juice.

4. Add in cooked sweet potatoes and black beans, toss with quinoa and stir to combine. Add in cilantro just before serving.

5. To serve, spoon sweet potato

Ingredients

1 tbsp olive oil and more for drizzling

½ red onion

2 cloves garlic, sliced

2 medium sweet potatoes, peeled and diced

1 can black beans, drained and rinsed

¼ cup cilantro

Juice of ½ lime

2 avocados

1½ tsp ground cumin

¼ tsp chili powder

1 bunch of collard greens or romaine lettuce hearts

½ tsp Celtic salt and more to taste

½ cup cooked quinoa or brown rice

mixture into a romaine lettuce cup or collard wrap. Top with avocado and salsa and serve!

Day 18

Learn To Cook

Learning to cook is one of the most important skills when creating a healthy lifestyle. It not only puts you in better control of what goes into your body, but also plays a key role in preventing boredom (one of the most common reasons why diets fail).

The idea behind learning to cook is not that you have to become a professional chef but instead, it simply encourages you to learn some key techniques to create delicious and healthy dishes at home. This starts with learning to appreciate the natural flavors of food and then focusing on bringing out the best in each ingredient instead of trying to mask the taste.

Also, try to simplify your cooking. You don't need thirty ingredients for a single dish. Look for recipes with around five ingredients and learn to actually prepare the lead ingredient so in the future, you can use what you have on hand and not have to worry about strictly following recipes.

So make the commitment to try one or two new recipes a week, paying special attention to flavor profiles you enjoy. Learn to season to your preferences and taste as you go, rather than waiting until the end and trying to fix it from there.

And don't be afraid to screw up! Making mistakes is how we learn but if you do find that your dish is lacking, try a squeeze of fresh lemon, a little hot sauce, a drizzle of olive oil or a pinch of Celtic salt to give it the kick of flavor it needs!

While learning to cook can take time, one tip that will change your cooking is to pick up some Celtic sea salt. It is a mineral-rich, coarse ground sea salt that will totally transform your cooking and add amazing flavor to your dishes without any extra effort. Just remember to taste as you cook as a little Celtic salt goes a long way.

Here's Your Game Plan For Day 18!

Continue your healthy habit and start your day as you mean to continue with some lemon water and a healthy breakfast!

Plan a hike. Take your body outdoors and explore the beautiful scenery around you while moving your body.

Breakfast: Day 18

Fix some savory oats with olive oil and Celtic salt and top with a hard-boiled egg to bump up the protein!

Lunch: Day 18

Toss some millet into the rice cooker – it's a delicious gluten free grain.

Dinner: Day 18

Tonight for dinner we're keeping it super simple with some roasted fish and veggies. Master this technique and you can prepare hundreds of variations of this meal at home! Recipes on pages 224-225.

Self Care

Go out and do something fun! Think of one thing you've been dying to do and go do it, no excuses. When we make it a priority to have fun and enjoy life, we're less likely to depend on food to fill a void.

Plan a small dinner party and share the new veggies you've been enjoying! #liveitshareit

Lemon Rosemary Salmon

1. Combine lemon juice, olive oil, rosemary, salt, red pepper and garlic. Brush mixture onto fish.

2. Arrange the fish on a baking sheet or broiling pan. Broil for 4-6 minutes per ½ inch of thickness until cooked through. If fish is more than 1 inch thick, gently turn it halfway through broiling.

Ingredients

4 pieces of salmon

1 tbsp olive oil

2 tsp fresh lemon juice

2 tsp fresh, chopped rosemary

2 cloves garlic, sliced

Celtic salt and red pepper to taste

3. Serve with green beans and mixed greens.

Green Beans With Rosemary

1. Preheat oven to 475 degrees. Toss all ingredients into a bowl and season with Celtic salt and red pepper flakes.

2. Spread on rimmed baking sheet. Roast 15-17 minutes, or until beans are tender and browned in spots, stirring occasionally.

Ingredients

1¼ lb green beans, trimmed

½ cup chopped walnuts

1½ tbsp finely chopped fresh rosemary

1 tbsp olive oil

Celtic salt

Red pepper flakes

Day 19

Clean Out Your Cupboards

Now that we're learning to cook and eating a variety of plant-based foods, it's time to clean out our cupboards and get rid of all those icky ingredients that are no longer serving us. In a perfect world, we would cook everything from scratch and stay away from packaged foods but for most of us, that's not realistic (although canned beans are a total lifesaver in my house for a quick source of protein). The key here is striving for progress, not perfection, and learning to choose better options when we can.

So today, let's focus on getting rid of any foods with long ingredient lists (most boxed cereals, granola bars, and boxed popcorn), artificial sugar (low-sugar yogurt, jams, and chewing gum), high fructose corn syrup (several breads, ketchup, and salad dressings), hydrogenated oils (peanut butter, non-dairy coffee creamers, and margarine), anything you can't pronounce, and foods that are overly processed (boxed mashed potatoes).

Fill your pantry instead with staples such as dried or organic canned beans, jarred tomatoes, gluten-free grains, minimally processed crackers and granola bars, canned sardines, herbs and spices, nut and seed butters, and healthy oils (coconut, grape seed, olive oil, and sesame oil) to make dinner at home convenient and easy.

And the same goes for your refrigerator and freezer – get rid of all of those convenience meals and check the labels on your condiments for hidden ingredients and excess sugar!

Here's Your Game Plan For Day 19!

It feels like another good day for your lemon water and breakfast combo!

Clean your house. It's a great way to get rid of clutter, leaving you

renewed and refreshed while also burning some extra calories. Crank up some music and dedicate one hour to tossing, donating, scrubbing, and simplifying your life.

Breakfast: Day 19

Bake up some sweet potatoes the night before and leave them on the counter. While you're getting ready, pop them in the oven to reheat and top off with some coconut butter or grass-fed butter and salt.

Lunch: Day 19

Looking for lunch out? Try sushi from your local health food store. Avocado rolls are my absolute favorite! Just make sure to skip all of the fancy sauces and stick to veggie or fish.

Dinner: Day 19

Make this quinoa salad for dinner tonight. It makes excellent leftovers and is best served over arugula or mixed greens! Need a little extra protein? Add some roasted chicken or a fried egg alongside. Bulk things up if you like! Turn to page 231.

Self Care

Put your fork down in between every bite and don't be afraid to leave food on your plate! Today, I want you to slow down between bites and pay more attention to the food in your mouth than the food on your fork. You'll find that you can better taste the food, and over time, you'll start to eat less. You may also feel some stress come up but that's normal. Explore how this new habit feels to you.

Post a photo on Instagram of all the crap you're throwing away! #liveitshareit

Herbed Quinoa And White Beans

1. Bring water to a boil and add quinoa. Reduce heat and simmer for 10-15 minutes until water has been absorbed. Alternatively, use a rice cooker.

2. In the meantime, sauté red onion in 1 tbsp olive oil and a pinch of salt for about 2 minutes. Add in asparagus and garlic and cook for another 5-6 minutes until softened. Stir in drained and rinsed beans and cook until heated through.

3. Check on quinoa after about 10 minutes and if water is mostly evaporated turn off heat and let sit for about 5-8 more minutes.

Ingredients

1 cup quinoa

1½ cups water or vegetable stock

1 tbsp olive oil for skillet and 3 tbsp more for dressing

Juice and zest of 1 lemon

¾ cup chopped basil

¼ cup chopped parsley

½ tbsp fresh thyme

1 bunch asparagus

1 small red onion

2 cloves garlic, sliced

2 cups of white beans

½ tsp Celtic sea salt

¼ tsp red pepper flakes

White balsamic (optional)

4. To prepare dressing, whisk together lemon juice, olive oil, and lemon zest before stirring in fresh herbs and salt to taste. Add

fluffed quinoa and bean mixture, toss to combine and top with a drizzle of white balsamic, black pepper, and Celtic salt. Serve room temperature, warm, or chilled! Serves 4-6.

Day 20

Learn To Prep Ahead

One thing I hear all the time from people is that they resort to fast or convenience foods because they didn't have the time to prepare or eat a healthy meal. While I totally understand that this happens from time to time, it's important when creating your healthy lifestyle to learn how to prepare for those busy days so you're not stuck in line at the drive-thru.

My biggest tip, and the most obvious for prepping ahead, is to always make extra when you do cook so you have at least one additional meal. It is one simple step that can make a huge difference. I often combine my leftovers with a big bed of greens for lunch with some hummus and crackers – it's filling and delicious!

Another way to make sure you always have healthy food on hand is to plan a day or two each week when you can do some batch cooking and either cut and prep or cook several days worth of food so all you have to do is come home and reheat.

Finally, choose some staples you enjoy to always keep on hand so you have no excuses when hunger strikes. For me, they're hard-boiled eggs, hummus and crackers, raw veggies, apples and almond butter, cooked quinoa with some Celtic salt and olive oil, or roasted veggies with some mustard and hot sauce.. This is one of the most difficult habits to form but once it becomes part of your weekly routine, healthy eating becomes easy and sustainable.

Here's Your Game Plan For Day 20!

Upon rising, start your day off with a mug of warm water with the juice of half a lemon and a small pinch of cayenne pepper. Sip that down followed by a cup of tea and then breakfast.

Dance! Put on your favorite song, let loose, and just dance!

Breakfast: Day 20

Crack an egg into an avocado half, season and bake at 425 degrees for 15-20 minutes or until egg is set. Top with some salsa and serve over a bed of arugula.

Lunch: Day 20

Roast a sweet potato and serve with black beans, massaged kale, and avocado.

Dinner: Day 20

Cook up a big pot of veggie chili – it's total comfort food and makes for great leftovers! Turn to page 237.

Self Care

Plan a fun night out with friends. This action gives you permission to just let go and have fun. The more fun you have in your life, the less you will rely on food to make you happy.

Invite a friend to come over and prep for the week together. Trade a few dishes! #liveitshareit

Vegetarian Chili

1. Sauté onions, carrots, peppers, and celery in olive oil with a pinch of salt and red pepper for about 10 minutes, or until tender. Stir in garlic, jalapeno, cumin, coriander, chili powder, cinnamon, and brown sugar and cook for another five minutes.

2. Add in vegetable stock cube, chipotle chilies, tomato sauce, water, and rice. Bring to a boil and reduce to a simmer, stirring in beans and soy sauce.

3. Simmer for at least one hour and up to three, adding more liquid as needed. (The chili could also be moved to a crock-pot at this point and cooked until desired thickness is reached).

Ingredients

1 tbsp olive oil

1 small red onion, diced

4 carrots, diced

2 celery stalks, diced

4 cloves garlic, sliced

2 bell peppers, diced (1 green and 1 red)

1 jalapeno pepper, seeds removed and diced

1 vegetable stock cube and 5 cups water

1 can tomato sauce

1 tsp cumin

1 tsp coriander

1 tsp Ancho chili powder

½ tsp cinnamon

2 tsp brown sugar

2½ tbsp soy sauce

3 chipotle chilies in adobo

½ cup short grain brown

4. Serve with green onion, a drizzle of olive oil, and pinch of salt!

rice

4 cups red beans, cooked

½ tsp Celtic salt

¼ tsp red pepper flakes

Day 21

Start Your Day Off Right

We're at day 21 and with just a week of guidance left, it's time to start creating some habits that will set you up for success. One of my favorites, and something that I believe has the opportunity to completely change your entire day, is the habit of starting your day off right.

Now it's not what you do that makes a difference, but rather starting your day in a way that will set you up for victory. So many women I know literally leave themselves just enough time to get out the door in the morning. This leads to stress, with crappy-breakfast-in-a-hurry resulting in less-than-stellar digestion, lack of enjoyment, and low energy, which just piles on even more stress!

Instead, I recommend taking just 30 minutes for yourself in the morning to create a ritual that will keep you relaxed and ready to handle any stress that comes your way. For me it's 15 minutes of gratitude/meditation/hot lemon water and then a healthy breakfast with a cup of tea that I genuinely enjoy before I do anything else.

Also, I have found that taking a step for your health first thing in the morning, such as lemon water and a good breakfast, really starts your morning off on a positive note and leads to better decision making for the rest of the day.

Here's Your Game Plan For Day 21!

I just mentioned it three lines ago and on day 21, you should need no reminders on how to start your day off right!

Invite a friend to go for a walk. Who says you can't socialize and sweat at the same time?

Breakfast: Day 21

Fix your favorite breakfast from what you've tried so far.

Lunch: Day 21

Take your leftover chili and stir some spinach into it because by now, you freaking love greens, right?

Dinner: Day 21

Keep it super simple tonight – roast up a bunch of veggies such as beets, Brussels sprouts, purple potato, carrot, parsnip, and onion. I like to combine all of my uniformly diced veggies on a baking sheet with some olive oil, Celtic salt, and herbs de Provence or fresh thyme and just roast at 425 degrees until tender and lightly browned. Serve with some pork, chicken, fish, or beans over some mixed greens or spinach.

Self Care

Buy yourself a new outfit that you look and feel

absolutely fabulous in!

Instagram a photo of your morning ritual. #liveitshareit

Day 22

Chew Your Food

The last time you had something to eat, did you give any thought to how long you chewed? For most people, chewing is done out of habit and as soon as a piece of food enters their mouths, they chew and swallow pretty quickly (especially when in a hurry or eating on the run as seems to be the case with so many people these days).

The chewing process is actually so important and serves as the first step in your digestive process. I'm a big advocate of properly chewing your food, as well as being aware of how much you chew, as it can significantly impact your health in ways you probably never knew!

First of all, and most importantly, chewing your food causes you to slow down and actually enjoy your meal. This prevents over-indulging and creates more pleasure from the experience of eating as you are better able to taste each bite.

Secondly, chewing your food enables you to get more nutrients from what you consume.

And finally, chewing helps ease the digestion process. Digestion is actually a very demanding task for your body and requires a great deal of energy, especially if forced to process improperly chewed food. Chewing properly allows your stomach to work more efficiently and break down your food faster. So today, make sure to put your fork down in between bites and make a conscious effort to chew each bite as well as you possibly can.

Here's Your Game Plan For Day 22!

Start YOUR day off right!

Do 25 push-ups – you can do the girl kind if you have to but try for the real ones

if possible!

Breakfast: Day 22

Cook up some old fashioned oats in water and serve drizzled with good olive oil, a pinch of Celtic salt, and red pepper flakes!

Lunch: Day 22

Asparagus soup is one of those things I look forward to each spring. It's super light and fresh, but loaded with fiber to keep me full and energized! Turn to page 247.

Dinner: Day 22

Veggie burgers are your best friend for quick and easy lunches and dinners. Make up a big ol' batch of these and either keep them in the fridge (for up to one week) or frozen (for up to three months) for a fabulous meal in minutes. Turn to page 248.

Self Care

Say No! Most of the women I work with do so much for others and rarely take time for themselves. Today I want you to choose one commitment that you don't really want to do and simply say, "No!" I know it's hard, but you will feel soooo good.

Take a date out for a nice dinner. Enjoy the experience and slow down. #liveitshareit

Farmers' Market Asparagus Soup

1. Bring water to a simmer in a large sauce pot and stir in vegetable stock cube to dissolve.

2. In a small skillet, sauté onion and leek in oil and ½ tsp salt until translucent, about 8 minutes.

3. In the meantime, dice asparagus and potato into small pieces, add to simmering water, cover and cook for 15 minutes, until tender.

Ingredients

1 bunch asparagus

2 red potatoes, peeled

4 cups water

1 vegetable stock cube

1 small leek

¼ yellow onion

1 tbsp olive oil

1 tsp Celtic salt

2 tbsp fresh basil

Pepper to taste

4. Add onions to the pot and ladle mixture into a blender. Purée in batches until smooth.

5. Add the remaining salt and pepper to taste, serve with a drizzle of olive oil and fresh basil!

Portobello Mushroom And Kale Burgers

1. Heat olive oil in a large pan over medium heat. Add in onion and sauté for about five minutes, or until tender. Dice up mushrooms and stir in with garlic. Cook until mushrooms become soft for 5-8 minutes. Stir in kale and cook another minute to wilt the kale. Remove pan from heat and set aside.

2. In a food processor, add oats and pulse a few times before adding ¾ of the mushroom mixture and the rest of the ingredients. Pulse mixture a few times until a "dough" forms, stir in remaining mixture and form into patties.

Ingredients

8 -10 oz baby bella mushrooms

1 small yellow onion, diced

4 stalks of kale, chopped

2 cloves garlic

1 tbsp olive oil

1½ tbsp tahini*

1 tbsp miso

½ tbsp tamari

1 cup oats

1 tsp vegan Worcestershire sauce

⅓ cup walnuts, toasted

½ tsp sage

1 tsp oregano

¼ cup fresh parsley

3. Cook in a skillet coated with olive oil over medium heat for about

four minutes per side. To grill, refrigerate at least an hour ahead of time!

4. Serve over a bed of spinach with baked sweet potato French fries

* Tahini or sesame paste can be found at your local ethnic market, health food store, or made at home by simply processing sesame seeds in the food processer until creamy.

Day 23

Breathe

Breathing is a simple practice to help you become present in the moment while cleansing the lymph system and improving your overall health. So many of us race through each day without actually enjoying what we're doing or eating. By slowing down and connecting with our breath on a regular basis, we become more connected with our body and its needs.

Set a timer on your phone multiple times throughout the day as a reminder to stop what you're doing and just breathe. My favorite breathing exercise to combat stress and center myself is to simply take three short inhalations followed by one long exhalation. I typically do this 5-6 times and find my whole body becomes relaxed and ready to take on whatever comes next!

I also practice taking a few deep breaths when I'm stressed, before eating, and for 10-20 minutes first thing in the morning to start my day off right and set me up for success throughout the day.

Here's Your Game Plan For Day 23!

Breathing isn't the only way to start your day off right – lemon water and a good breakfast will help too!

Try kettlebells – they're a great way to get a total body workout and raise your heart rate in minutes.

Breakfast: Day 23

Chia pudding is another one of my favorites for breakfast on the run. I like to use the basic formula and then change up my toppings with the seasons. My absolute favorite way to serve this however is with some fresh blueberries and walnuts and if I'm really hungry, I serve a hard-boiled egg alongside. Turn to page 254.

Lunch: Day 23

Leftover veggie burgers in romaine lettuce heart cups and raw veggies and hummus make lunch a breeze!

Dinner: Day 23

Got the urge to dine out? Try Chipotle as a great, healthy fast food option. I love the fact that they source local ingredients where possible and prepare most of their foods from scratch! Just steer clear of cheese, sour cream, and tortillas and don't eat the entire thing!

Self Care

Take 10 minutes today and meditate. It doesn't have to be perfect, but taking the time to clear your mind and focus on your breath can have a huge impact on mindfulness and stress management throughout the day!

Tweet about what you did to just breathe. #liveitshareit

Vanilla Chia Pudding

1. Combine all of the ingredients in a blender, and blend until a uniform texture is achieved. Alternatively, whisk together in a glass bowl.

2. Transfer to a sealed container and allow to chill at least three hours to overnight. Serves one.

Ingredients

3 tablespoons chia seeds

1 cup almond milk

1 teaspoon vanilla extract

1 tablespoon pure maple syrup or 1 date

Day 24

Focus On Enjoying Your Life Now, Not 20 lbs From Now

One thing I hear ALL the time from so many women is that they will be happy, accomplish goals, and enjoy life when they are thin. In fact, I think a lot of people think this way and it breaks my heart to hear this mindset. Even worse, the truth is that they couldn't possibly be more wrong.

Thinking that you're unhappy because you're overweight and in turn punishing yourself with strict diet and exercise to remedy that issue will only lead to tension in your body and sabotage your efforts.

Think about it this way – any type of stress (even emotional) causes the body to enter into a state of protection, also known as "fight or flight." This results in altered hormone levels as the body shuts down all processes not directly required for survival. Part of the stress response, as stated above, is the release of cortisol, which holds onto fat for protection. So when you're in a constant state of hating your body, you'll never reach your goals no matter how hard you try because your body is inherently protecting you.

Instead, make the choice to be happy. Striving toward the way you want to feel will increase chemical neurotransmitters sometimes called happy hormones. This starts the process of balancing your hormones, which will help your body release unnecessary weight.

Have fun every day and focus on small steps to help you reach your goals and just do the best you can. If you want a cookie, have it, and enjoy every bite, but remember to nourish your body with as many nutrient-dense foods as you can the rest of the day. Over time you will get to that ideal weight for your body and enjoy the process much more along the way.

Here's Your Game Plan For Day 24!

Upon rising, start your day off with a mug of warm water with the juice of half a lemon and a small pinch of cayenne pepper. Sip that down followed by a cup of tea and then breakfast.

Get outside – hike, bike, walk, anything to soak up a little vitamin D and move your body in a way you enjoy!

Breakfast: Day 24

Delicious and creamy, my pomegranate-ginger smoothie is the perfect way to start your day! Turn to page 259.

Lunch: Day 24

I love to repurpose leftovers throughout the week so I never get bored. Serve this soup over rice or cooked spaghetti squash to switch things up! Turn to page 260.

Dinner: Day 24

Quinoa salads are a staple in my house – I love to make up a big batch at the beginning of the week and then add them to my meals all week long. Use this recipe as a template and switch up the vegetables as the seasons change. Turn to page 261.

Self Care

Soak in nature – embrace the beauty surrounding you! I love to find a local arboretum or park and just appreciate all the gorgeousness nature has to offer!

Post a photo on Instagram of you doing something fun today! #liveitshareit

Pomegranate-Ginger Smoothie

1. Blend all ingredients in a high speed blender until smooth. Enjoy immediately.

Ingredients

Seeds and juice from one pomegranate

1 granny smith apple, cored

1 handful spinach

¼-½ of an avocado

½ inch knob of fresh ginger, peeled

1 cup non-dairy milk (unsweetened)

Handful of ice

Creamy Roasted Tomato Soup

1. Preheat oven to 375 degrees. Halve tomatoes and place on a baking sheet with garlic head. Drizzle liberally with olive oil and season with Celtic salt, red pepper, and herbs de Provence.

2. Bake for 30-45 minutes until garlic begins to brown and tomatoes are fragrant and tender.

3. Peel tomato skins from tomatoes, pop out garlic cloves, and add both to a blender with sugar, balsamic, stock cube, and water.

4. Blend until smooth and transfer to a saucepan to warm. To serve drizzle with olive oil and season to taste with Celtic salt and red pepper.

Ingredients

2 lbs roma tomatoes

½ tsp herbs de Provence

1 head garlic, top removed

¼ tsp Celtic salt

red pepper flakes

olive oil

½ tbsp sugar

1 tsp balsamic vinegar

½ vegetable stock cube

½ cup water

Roasted Summer Vegetable And Quinoa Salad

1. Preheat the oven to 425 degrees. In a bowl, combine all of the cubed veggies and toss with the herbs de Provence, garlic, oil and salt. Place in a single layer on a lined baking sheet and bake for 30 minutes, flipping half way through. I usually flip to broil the last few minutes to brown things up!

2. Add quinoa and stock to a rice cooker and cook until fluffy. In a glass bowl, combine cooked quinoa with roasted veggies. Add dressing, toss and enjoy hot, room temperature or cold (4-6 servings). Serve over mixed greens!

Ingredients

1 cup quinoa

1½ cups vegetable stock

1 tsp extra virgin olive oil

4 cloves garlic, sliced

½ tsp Celtic salt

2 bell peppers, cubed

1 zucchini, cubed

1 red onion, cubed

1 fennel bulb, cubed

1 tsp herbs de Provence

For the dressing:

2 tbsp extra virgin olive oil

½ tsp Celtic salt

½ lemon, juiced and zested

Fresh herbs – basil, parsley (optional)

Day 25

Keep Portions In Check: What Portion Control Looks Like

Although I am not at all a fan of calorie counting or obsession over what goes into your mouth on a daily basis, I do believe awareness is key to sustainable weight loss and maintenance. With that in mind, I think it's important to understand what a proper portion looks like.

Our current culture is so absorbed in getting value for our money that we have completely lost the concept of satiety and instead, we end up eating beyond oblivion. This is detrimental to our health for two reasons. Firstly, this behavior causes us to lose all awareness and pleasure in our food, and secondly, we consistently overeat for no reason at all, putting excess stress on our body as we try to digest all of that food we don't really need.

To curb these habits, I believe that we must be aware of what a proper portion entails and become mindful as we eat so overdoing our food intake becomes less of a habit.

Think of it this way: 1 portion = 1 medium apple

Since it's so important to listen to your body and eat what you need each day, I think it's less significant to get fixated on how many portions you consume. A better approach is to focus on the fact that you had two portions of chicken (because you needed it) and 4 portions of kale (because you were hungry). The idea is to have reasons for what you eat, not excuses.

Awareness and mindfulness are key so when you sit down to a meal, get in tune with how hungry you are, slow down as you eat, and recognize when you've had enough. It may seem like a difficult practice at first but once you get the hang of things, intuitive eating will become habit and you'll be surprised how much less food your body really needs.

And remember, when you feel the desire to overdo it, take a step back, breathe, and remember you WILL eat again.

Here's Your Game Plan For Day 25!

Make it a priority to start your day off right!

Take a new fitness class – try Zumba or kickboxing with a girlfriend. Who knows, you might find a new favorite way to move your body!

Breakfast: Day 25

Cook some of my favorite Love Grown Super Oats and top off with some apple slices, cinnamon, coconut oil, and a touch of maple syrup!

Lunch: Day 25

Time for that leftover quinoa salad. Add a small portion of chicken or fish for extra protein if needed!

Dinner: Day 25

This soup is another one of those recipes where once you learn the technique you can use what you have on hand. I love swapping out the white potato for sweet potato in this one or using white beans instead of black-eyed peas! Herbs de Provence also makes a great alternative if you don't have fresh herbs on hand. Turn to page 266.

Self Care

Smile at yourself. You are amazing.

Have a tapas party and share what you learned about portions! #liveitshareit

Black Eyed Pea And Kale Soup

1. Heat oil in a large pot over medium heat. Add onions and a pinch of salt. Sauté for 2-3 minutes until the onions begin to soften before adding in potato and carrots. Cook together for another 8-10 minutes until veggies begin to become tender and start to cook through.

2. Stir in rosemary, mushrooms, tomatoes, thyme, garlic, a pinch of red pepper, black-eyed peas, vegetable stock cube, and enough water to cover.

3. Bring pot to a boil and reduce to a simmer for 15-20 minutes until everything is tender, stir in kale and cook another 3-4 minutes until kale is wilted. Adjust seasonings and top with a

Ingredients

2 cups black eyed peas

1 tbsp olive oil

1 small yellow onion

2 carrots, sliced

1 Yukon gold potato, cut into small cubes

6 cloves garlic, sliced

1 sprig rosemary (1tsp)

3 sprigs fresh thyme (1 tsp)

1 8oz can diced tomatoes

1 vegetable stock cube

Enough water to cover veggies

4 kale leaves, cut into ribbons

½ tsp Celtic salt, to taste

¼-½ tsp red pepper flakes

4 dried shitake mushrooms, sliced

drizzle of olive oil and a pinch of salt to serve.

Day 26

Incorporate Probiotic Rich Foods

For the past twenty-five days, we've been building the foundation for a long-term, sustainably healthy lifestyle. Today, however, it's time to go a little deeper and talk about something that is absolutely essential in achieving optimal health and that I know has immensely improved my own.

Probiotics are the beneficial bacteria found in the gut that aid in improving the health of our intestines. Probiotics help to enhance the function of our immune systems (70% of our immune system is in our gut), while increasing the bio-availability of nutrients we get from the foods we eat.

Having the proper balance of gut bacteria and enough digestive enzymes helps you absorb nutrients while putting less stress on your digestive system, freeing up more energy for other things. This will play a tremendous role in decreased cravings since you're getting everything you need from the foods you're consuming.

Although supplementing probiotics is a good idea, I also highly recommend consuming probiotics in the form of food and drinks as well. Some of my favorite sources include kombucha, water kefir, sauerkraut, kimchi, fermented carrots and pickles, and kavass.

Here's Your Game Plan For Day 26!

How could you possibly start your day with anything other than warm lemon water, tea and breakfast?

Practice contracting your abs throughout the day. It's an easy way to work your core as well as focus on good posture, which

naturally makes you look younger and thinner

Breakfast: Day 26

Breakfast doesn't always have to be complicated. I often eat last night's leftovers for breakfast when I am not in the mood to cook anything fancy.

Lunch: Day 26

Leftover soup and a salad or serve leftover soup over rice and top with a fried egg!

Dinner: Day 26

Make your favorite tacos and serve them in romaine lettuce hearts instead of shells. My favorite combination includes black beans, quinoa, peppers and onions, fresh salsa, guacamole, and cilantro.

Self Care

Read a good book. Allow yourself the opportunity to let go of all of the things on your to-do list and instead focus on getting lost in a good book. Just an hour of time for yourself can make all the difference in increasing your productivity when it's time to get back to reality.

Share a kombucha with your best friend! #liveitshareit

Day 27

Shift Your Mindset: Focus On Becoming Better Than You Were The Day Before

As we wind down with the last few days of this program, it's important to continue to focus on the habits that you've been cultivating this month and to remember that creating a healthy lifestyle is about taking things one day at a time. If you do more than that, you'll find yourself overwhelmed.

And when you have a bad day, don't stress out or get angry and beat yourself up – instead focus on getting back on track. Stop, breathe, practice self-love, move a little more, eat a little less and remember that it's all about the journey. Focus on the simple act of making a conscious effort to do something for your health each and every day and try to be better than you were the day before. It's that simple and with this mindset, you'll never fail. And if you don't believe me, I know from experience that taking things one day at a time is the only way to truly enjoy the process and get where you want to go.

Here's Your Game Plan For Day 27!

Upon rising, start your day off with a mug of warm water with the juice of half a lemon and a small pinch of cayenne pepper. Sip that down followed by a cup of tea and then breakfast.

Try yoga before bed. It's a great way to unwind and induce better sleep.

Breakfast: Day 27

Tamago Kake Gohan is one of those traditional Japanese inspired dishes that's insanely simple but so rich and flavorful at the same time. If you're not comfortable with the raw egg, simply fry up the eggs and add the mirin and soy sauce in the skillet to finish. Don't skip the nori, it's surprisingly delicious as it softens due to the warm rice. Turn to page 276.

Lunch: Day 27

Choose your favorite – just make sure it includes some leafy greens!

Dinner: Day 27

I came up with this chickpea curry recipe back in college when I only had 30 minutes to cook on any given night. I recommend using a rice cooker for the rice to speed up and simplify the process. And don't be afraid to serve the curry room temp over some mixed greens for lunch – it's delicious! Turn to page 277.

Self Care

Read beauty product labels. By now, we're feeding ourselves well so let's focus on taking care of our body in the best way possible.

Our skin is our largest organ so what we put on it goes directly into our blood stream. I love using coconut oil as a moisturizer for my body and washing my face with honey in the morning and a combo of olive oil and castor oil at night. Take things one day at a time – simple swaps add up!

Share one thing you want to do for your health on Twitter. #liveitshareit

Tamago Kake Gohan

1. Rinse your uncooked rice until the water is clear. Cook rice in a rice cooker or in a pot over medium heat (½ cup rice to 1 cup water). Place in bowl.

2. Take raw egg and mix with soy sauce. Mirin is optional and adds a light sweetness to the dish.

Ingredients

½ cup Japanese rice

1 cup water

2 Eggs

1 tbsp soy sauce

1 tsp mirin

Furikake (nori)

Green onion

Whisk. Pour over rice. Top with furikake and green onion. Serves two.

**If you're not a fan of raw egg mix the soy/mirin mixture with the rice and top off with a fried egg and nori to serve.

Chickpea Curry In A Hurry

1. Bring water to a boil in a large pan. Add rice, reduce to a simmer and cook 45-50 minutes.

2. Heat the oil in a large pan. Add the onion and garlic and cook until the onion is tender, about 5-7 minutes. Add the curry and ginger and cook until fragrant, about one minute. Add the tomatoes, hot sauce, chickpeas and water and bring to a boil.

3. Reduce the heat and simmer covered for about 10-15 minutes, stir in spinach to wilt. Serve over brown rice and garnish with fresh cilantro!

Ingredients

2 cups water

1 cup brown rice

1 tbsp oil

1 onion (chopped)

2 tbsp curry powder

2 cloves garlic, sliced

1 tbsp fresh ginger, minced

1 14 oz can diced tomatoes

2 tsp hot sauce

1 can chickpeas (rinsed and drained)

1 cup water or coconut milk

Celtic salt to taste

¼ cup cilantro (chopped)

1 cup spinach cut into ribbons

Day 28

Find Passion In Your Healthy Lifestyle

I am a strong believer that when you're truly passionate about something, you will have the greatest success. When we are passionate about an activity, we naturally put more effort into it, have more energy towards it, and find creativity to keep things exciting. I was lucky to discover my passion for food, health, and nutrition at a young age, but I am always amazed to watch women as they discover their passions while creating their own healthy lifestyles.

So today, I want you to find your passion. Whatever it may be, find the one thing about this lifestyle you're creating that truly lights you up. It might be trying new recipes, spending time at the farmers' market, greens, discovering new cuisines, yoga, meditation, spinning, gratitude journaling, sharing food with others, talking about your experiences, healthy menu planning, or your daily walk with a friend. Finding that passion is key to sustaining this lifestyle in the long term as passion will help to keep you going and get you back on track when you hit bumps along the way.

To create a deeper bond, I suggest sharing your passion on social media with the hash tag *#liveitshareit* and connect with the like-minded people around you, sharing their love for the lifestyle they've created.

Here's Your Game Plan For Day 28!

How did you ever start the day without lemon water and a healthy breakfast?

Search on YouTube for a quick booty workout and spend at least 10 minutes

strengthening your tush!

Breakfast: Day 28

Tofu scrambles are a fun alternative to eggs and make the perfect weekend brunch when served alongside some sweet potato hash and sautéed kale! If you're not a tofu fan, simply sub in a few scrambled eggs! Turn to page 282.

Lunch: Day 28

Make a big salad with quinoa, roasted veggies, and hummus. For a little extra protein, top off with some canned sardines!

Dinner: Day 28

I love this soup. It's extremely simple yet rich in flavors. If you're looking to bulk things up add some white fish on top and then broil until cooked through. Turn to page 283.

Self Care

Put your phone down! So much of our lives are consumed by technology that we often don't notice we're even using it. Today, leave your phone in your purse during meals, don't check it at every stop light, and after 9pm, turn it off for a good night's sleep!

Set an example and inspire others by sharing what you learn. Create support and accountability for yourself! #liveitshareit

Jamaican Curried Tofu Scramble

1. Add water and vegetable stock cube to a skillet over medium heat. Cook to dissolve cube, add onions and sauté for 5 minutes until they begin to soften.

2. In the meantime, press water out of tofu, crumble and set aside. Add garlic to skillet followed by tofu and tomatoes and cook for another 5 minutes before adding in curry, nutritional yeast, salt, and red pepper.

3. Cook until well combined, stirring occasionally, and add in spinach just before serving and finish with a drizzle of olive oil and pinch of Celtic salt.

Ingredients

1 package firm tofu

¼ red onion

1 cup cherry tomatoes halved

2 cloves garlic, sliced

1 vegetable stock cube

2 tbsp water

¼ tsp Celtic salt

¼ tsp red pepper flakes

2 tbsp Jamaican curry powder

1 tbsp nutritional yeast

1 cup spinach, cut into ribbons

Caribbean Black Bean Soup

1. Combine ingredients except for cilantro and lime zest in a pie pan, pop into a preheated 500 degree oven and bake for 15 minutes until fragrant.

2. Top with fresh cilantro and lime zest before serving. Serves two.

Ingredients

1 can black beans, not drained

¼ cup beer

¾ tsp jerk seasoning

½ tbsp butter

1 large garlic clove

⅛ small red onion

¼ tsp Celtic sea salt

¼ tsp red pepper flakes

2 tbsp fresh cilantro

¼ lime, zested

Recipe Index

ACKNOWLEDGEMENTS

I want to thank:

My editor, Mike Ahern, who helped take my thoughts and shape them into an incredible story of which I am so proud. Without your help, this book might still be written on a napkin.

My Aunt Marilyn, who made healthy cooking fun and inspired me to grow up and share my passion for health and nutrition with the world.

Debbie Flynn. Growing up, I always wanted to be an entrepreneur just like you, helping and inspiring people to live a little healthier. I am so blessed to have you as an example in my life.

My sister Annie and brother-in-law David, my ultimate taste testers. David, I am thankful to know you'll happily try anything I cook and Annie, you have no idea how proud it makes me to see all of the amazing things you cook when I'm not around. Keep on eating those greens ;)

ABOUT THE AUTHOR

Meet Kate Horning: Health Coach. Lifestyle Expert. Chef.

Kate Horning is an emerging thought leader in health and nutrition. She is an ambassador on the leading edge of a new generation that challenges established ideas, looking for better ways to achieve healthier, happier lives.

Kate's journey began with a book report at age thirteen, to be allowed by her mother to become a vegetarian. That sparked a passion that has led to studying and living nutrition for over a decade. Through her personal experiments with the typical American diet, as a vegetarian, vegan, calorie counter, and raw foodie, she has discovered the secrets of developing a practical, sustainable, healthy lifestyle.

As a high school senior, Kate gave a keynote address on childhood obesity advising the state of Ohio's Board of Education on local school wellness policy. She is a supporter of fighting childhood obesity through health and nutrition education.

Kate studied dietetics at the University of Kentucky, and is a certified holistic health coach and chef.

Made in the USA
San Bernardino, CA
14 May 2014